Clinical Radiology

made
ridiculously
simple

Hugue Ouellette MD, FRCPC
Associate Program Director
Department of Radiology
Director of Education
Musculoskeletal Radiology
Massachusetts General Hospital
Harvard Medical School

Patrice Tétreault MD, FRCPC
Chief of Othopedic Surgery
Hôpital Notre-Dame du CHUM
University of Montréal

MedMaster, Inc. Miami

ISBN 978-0-940780-75-0

Made in the United States of America

Published by
MedMaster, Inc.
P.O. Box 640028
Miami FL 33164

A mes êtres les plus chers: Lise, Jean-Paul, Jeannette, Alcide et ma petite fleur.

Hugue Ouellette M.D.

A mes parents, Pierrette et Yvon.

Patrice Tétreault, M.D.

Acknowledgments

E. Stewart M.D.
J. Lin M.D. Ph.D.
A. Tremblay B.Sc.
M. Davis M.D.
C. Dennie M.D.
F. Matzinger M.D.
S. Grahovac M.D.
W. Morrish M.D.
H. Tao M.D.
B. Wong M.D.
C. Michaud M.D.
A. Lum M.D.
S. Millward M.D.
J. Aquino M.D.
P. Kalapos M.D.
T. Tebbenham M.D.
M. Chiu M.D.
S. Girard M.D.
R. Blumer M.D.
F. Lee M.D.
J. Yu M.D.
H. Hejjaji M.D.
L. Howlett M.D.
B. Sherlock
E. Fliszar
"Fisher" (our laptop computer)

CONTENTS

PREFACE

This book was written with the intention to pursue Dr. Stephen Goldberg's vision to make learning ridiculously simple. It is designed to rapidly teach the clinically vital components of radiology. The reader will acquire a solid approach to radiographic examinations commonly interpreted without radiologist assistance, and will become comfortable at recognizing common and dangerous conditions. Although this book is intended for medical students and interns, it is also useful for nurses, nurse practitioners and X-ray technicians.

This small text is not meant to be a synopsis of the broad field of radiology. Radiographic examinations interpreted by medical students and interns in the emergency room or on the ward are emphasized, while more advanced topics are ignored. For example, plain radiographs of the chest, abdomen and bones are discussed. Small chapters on the intravenous pyelogram and computed tomography (CT) of the head are also included. However, several topics such as barium studies, ultrasonography and magnetic resonance imaging (MRI) are underemphasized or completely ignored in the text, but presented in greater detail on the CD.

Each chapter is subdivided into Radiographic Anatomy, Approach and Specific Problem sections. In the Radiographic Anatomy sections, key anatomical landmarks are identified using simplified illustrations. In the Approach sections, reading of the radiographic examination is explained using analogies, illustrative cartoons and mnemonics. In the Specific Problem sections, the radiographic findings of the most common and deadly conditions are discussed.

Much of this book was written in the Greek islands, where "simplicity" is a way of life. We hope that simplicity is reflected in this work, and that you will have as much fun learning about radiology as we did writing about it.

Special thanks to Dr. Evelyn Stewart who was the first to believe in the project and who proof read the text countless times, to Dr. Jenny Lin, Ms. Annie Tremblay, our families and friends, the Radiology department at the University of Ottawa, and the Orthopedics department at the University of Montreal for their unconditional support. Also special thanks to Dr. Michael Davis, a truly inspirational teacher.

Y'a rien d'impossible!

Hugue Ouellette, M.D.
Patrice Tétreault, M.D.

Chapter 1.   The Basics

I. Plain x-ray film

Do the following small experiments. Turn on a desk lamp and hold your finger under it. The light represents the x-ray source while the desk is analogous to the film.

    Experiment 1:   Put a drinking glass beside your finger. Notice that the finger shadow is darker than the glass shadow because it is denser. X-ray shadows behave in much the same way. Radiographic film before an image is taken is transparent and therefore white on a view box. When a radiograph is taken, X-rays reach the film and darken it. The more X-rays reach an area of the film, the darker that area will be on the radiograph. Therefore, if an object is very dense, less X-rays will reach the film and consequently the image of the object will appear white on the radiograph. However, if an object has little density, its image will appear black on the radiograph because it allows most of the X-ray beam to reach the film.

Only five basic radiographic densities exist. They are in order of increasing brightness; *gas, fat, fluid, bone and metal densities.* This is a *key concept* (Fig.1-1). Anatomic structures seen on the radiograph can be identified by their characteristic density. For example, the lungs are dark, or air density, because they are filled with air. Organs such as the heart are largely composed of water. Therefore it is no surprise that they appear lighter than the lungs, because they are fluid density. Bones are brighter structures because they are composed of calcium.

    Experiment 2:   Put your finger near your desk. Notice how sharp the shadow is. Now move the finger away from your desk toward the light. Notice how the shadow becomes bigger and more blurred. Similarly, the closer an object is to the film, the sharper the borders are. The farther away from the film it is, the more magnified and fuzzy is the shadow of the object.

    Experiment 3:   Put your index fingers one against the other and observe the shadow they cast. The border between them cannot be seen. Therefore, when two structures of the same density are in anatomical contact with each other, the border between them cannot be seen. For example, if pneumonia (fluid density) is affecting the lung adjacent to the heart (also fluid density), the border or silhouette of the heart will not be seen.

II. CT scan and MRI

Imagine now that while you are doing the above experiments, the lamp and the desk start spinning rapidly around your finger. This situation is analogous to a *CT scan (Computed Tomography).* The x-ray tube and the detector spin rapidly around the patient. Information is transferred to a computer and multiple images are reconstructed. CT images give the impression of looking at cross-sectional slices of the patient. *MRI (Magnetic Resonance Imaging)* generates cross-sectional images using a large magnetic field. No x-rays are used.

III. General approach

Although there is a specific approach to each radiographic examination, the following principles hold true for all of them.

    A. Labels

There is nothing more embarrassing than making the right diagnosis on the wrong patient. One *must* always look at the label for the proper identification of the patient.

    B. Previous exams

If possible, have a previous exam for comparison. This is extremely important to determine if a problem is chronic (old) or acute (new).

1

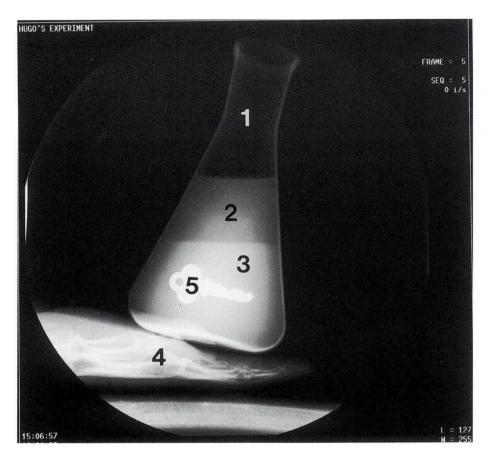

Fig.1-1: **Key concept.** The five radiographic densities are in order of increasing brightness: 1. Air, 2. Fat, 3. Fluid, 4. Bone, 5. Metal.

C. Quality of the film

A good quality film can really improve the precision of a diagnosis. A film should not be too dark (*over exposed;* Fig.1-2) or too white (*under exposed;* Fig.1-3). Also, assess if the patient is slightly turned to one side or the other when the film was taken.

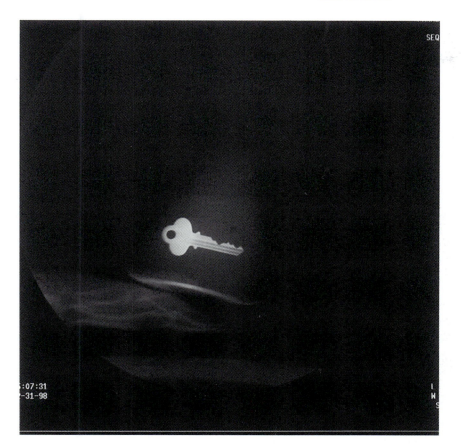

Fig.1-2: Over exposed film. The long exposure time results in a much darker film. The border between air and fat is lost.

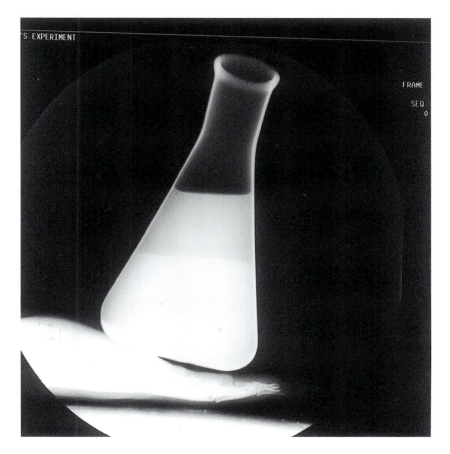

Fig.1-3: Under exposed film. The short exposure time results in a much brighter film. The border between the key and fluid is lost.

Chapter 2.   Chest Radiograph

I. Radiographic anatomy

A. Basic views

1. Posteroanterior view (PA view)

Remember that the closer an object is to the film, the sharper are the borders. The further away it is from the film, the more magnified and fuzzy is the shadow of the object (The Basics; experiment 2). Most of the important structures in the chest such as the heart and great vessels are located anteriorly. Therefore it is not surprising that the best way to take a chest radiograph is with the patient's front against the film. The X-ray is shot from the patient's back and is therefore called the posteroanterior view or PA view. On such a film, the heart size is minimally magnified and the heart borders are sharp (Fig.2-1AB).

2. Anteroposterior view (AP view)

Sometimes the patient is too sick to stand or sit for a PA view. In this case, a lower quality AP view is taken. A film is placed under the patient's back and an X-ray is shot through the patient from the front. In this view, the heart is farther from the film. Therefore, it appears larger than it really is and its borders are fuzzier, just like the finger in our experiment (The Basics; experiment 2).

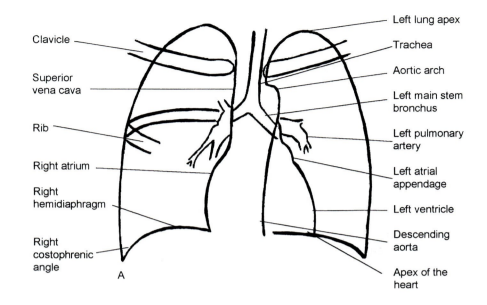

Clavicle

Superior vena cava

Rib

Right atrium

Right hemidiaphragm

Right costophrenic angle

Left lung apex

Trachea

Aortic arch

Left main stem bronchus

Left pulmonary artery

Left atrial appendage

Left ventricle

Descending aorta

Apex of the heart

A

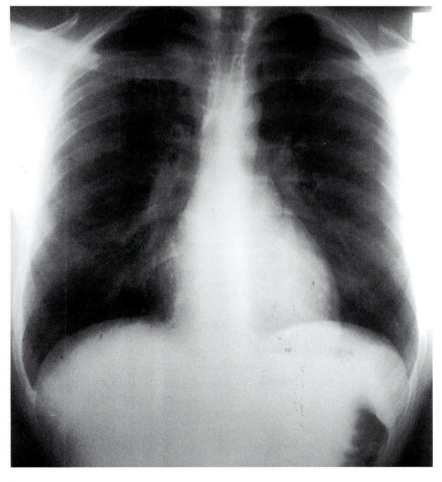

B

Fig.2-1: Normal chest radiographs. A. Diagram of a normal PA chest radiograph. B. Normal PA chest radiograph. C. Diagram of a normal lateral chest radiograph. D. Normal lateral chest radiograph.

3. Lateral view

The lateral view is taken with the patient in profile. It is taken routinely with the PA view to localize lung lesions, which may be hidden behind the heart or the diaphragm (Fig.2-1CD).

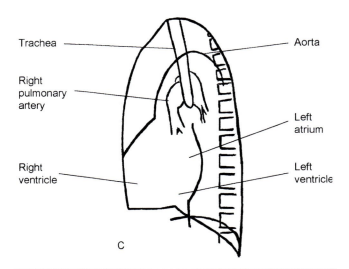

Trachea

Right pulmonary artery

Right ventricle

Aorta

Left atrium

Left ventricle

C

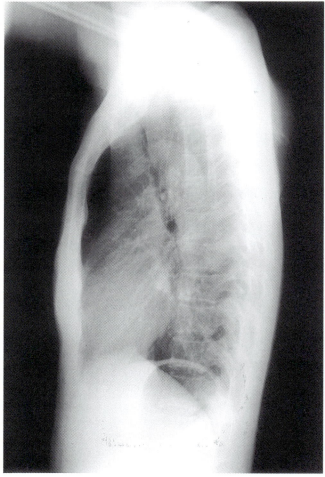

D

Fig.2-1   *(continued)*

4. Decubitus view

Decubitus is just a fancy Latin word for *lying down.* Therefore, this view is a PA view with the patient lying on his/her side. This view is useful to identify fluid in the pleural space. Fluid is heavier than air and always collects in the lowest portion of the chest due to gravity. For example, if a pleural effusion is suspected over the right hemidiaphragm, one should obtain a radiograph with the patient lying on the right side (right lateral decubitus view) to confirm the diagnosis. The fluid would then accumulate against the right chest wall.

B. Mediastinum

The mediastinum contains several important structures, including the heart, the great vessels, the trachea, the mainstem bronchi, the esophagus and innumerable lymph nodes. The mediastinum connects with each lung via a bridge-like structure called the *hilum.*

On a frontal (PA or AP) radiograph, the right mediastinal silhouette is composed of the superior vena cava and the right atrium. The left mediastinal silhoutte is composed of 3 major bumps, which represent the aortic arch, the left atrial appendage and the left ventricle/heart apex. In addition to the mediastinal silhouette, one can also see the right and left pulmonary arteries that extend from their respective hila and the descending aorta behind the heart. The trachea and mainstem bronchi are also well seen and have the appearance of a dark inverted Y over the heart (Fig.2-1AB).

On a lateral film, the anterior border of the heart is composed of the right ventricle, and the posterior border is composed of the left atrium superiorly and the left ventricle inferiorly. The dark trachea and the aorta are also well visualized behind the heart. The right pulmonary artery seen "head on", looks like a white thumb print and should be no larger than thumb-size (Fig.2-1CD).

C. Lungs/pleura

On a frontal radiograph of the lungs, the pulmonary arteries are seen branching out from the hila. Notice that the lower branches are larger due to the effect of gravity. Remember that bronchi in the lung are invisible on a normal radiograph because their walls are very thin, they contain air, and are surrounded by air.

The right lung is composed of 3 lobes called the upper, middle and lower lobes (Fig.2-2ABC). The left lung is composed of only 2 lobes, called the upper and lower lobes. The left equivalent of the right middle lobe (RML) is the *lingula,* a tongue-like portion of the left upper lobe that "licks" the left heart border. Lobes are separated from each other by fissures. In the right lung, the oblique fissure separates the lower lobe from the middle lobe, and the horizontal fissure separates the

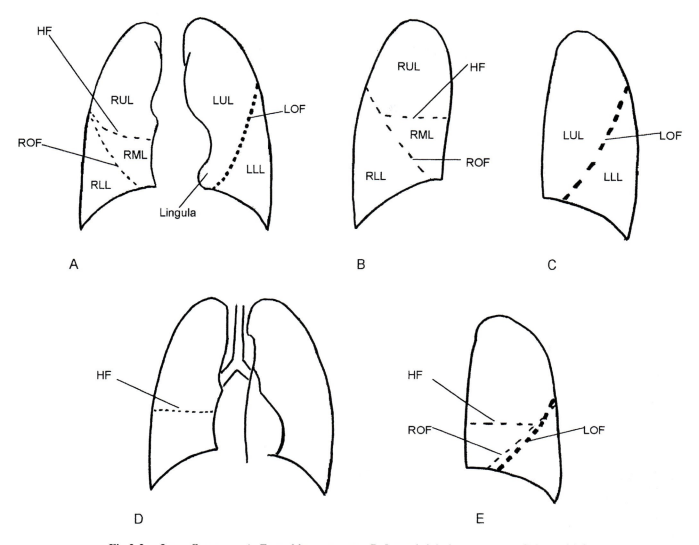

Fig.2-2: Lung fissures. A. Frontal lung anatomy. B. Lateral right lung anatomy. C. Lateral left lung anatomy. D. Drawing of the PA radiograph of the chest. The horizontal fissure (HF) of the right lung can be seen on this view. E. Drawing of the lateral chest radiograph. Both the superimposed oblique fissures and the horizontal fissure can be seen on the lateral view. Right upper lobe (RUL), right middle lobe (RML), right lower lobe (RLL), left upper lobe (LUL), left lower lobe (LLL), horizontal fissure (HF), right oblique fissure (ROF), left oblique fissure (LOF).

middle lobe from the upper lobe. In the left lung, a single oblique fissure separates the upper lobe from the lower lobe.

Each lobe is covered by a thin layer of tissue called visceral pleura. Fissures are composed of the visceral pleura of two adjacent lobes. Fissures are very thin structures that are only seen when parallel to the x-ray beam. Therefore, the horizontal (minor) fissure can be seen on both the PA view and the lateral view, while the oblique (major) fissures can only be seen on the lateral view (Fig. 2-2DE). There is also a thin layer of tissue covering the interior of the chest wall and the diaphragm, called the parietal pleura. The parietal pleura and the visceral pleura of the peripheral aspect of the lung are normally so close to each other that there is no real space between them. There is only a potential space between

them, although in certain disease states they may be separated by fluid or air (i.e. pleural effusion or pneumothorax, respectively).

The parietal pleura reflects deep into the recesses made by the diaphragm and the chest wall. These recesses are called anterior, lateral and posterior *costophrenic angles* or *sulci*. The one that extends most inferiorly is the posterior sulcus.

The *interstitium* is the scaffolding of the lung. It includes the interlobular septa with their vessels and lymphatics, the bronchi and pulmonary arterioles, and the very thin alveolar walls. The bronchi course through the lung and become smaller bronchioles, leading to clumps of "grape-like" structures called the *alveoli*. Each small clump of grapes, called a *lobule*, is separated by a soft tissue wall called the *interlobular septum*.

D. Chest wall

The chest wall is composed of ribs, muscle and fat. Remember that large breasts appear as diffuse white areas overlying the lower lungs. This may be incorrectly interpreted as the lungs being too white.

E. Diaphragm

The diaphragm is composed of the right and left *hemidiaphragm,* which are dome-like structures. On the frontal radiograph, notice that the right hemidiaphragm is higher than the left one because of the presence of the liver just under it. On the lateral radiograph, the heart sits on the left hemidiaphragm, which helps to differentiate it from the right one.

II. Approach

A. Basics

1. Marker

Verify that the marker is on the appropriate side of the heart (usually "L" for left). If the location of the apex of the heart and the "L" are on opposite sides, either the film was mislabeled or the patient's heart is on the wrong side (*dextrocardia*).

2. Inspiration

A deep inspiration is needed to obtain a good image of the lungs. If the lungs span 9 ribs, the inspiration is adequate.

3. Exposure

Assess the film's exposure. If the spine cannot be seen behind the heart, the film is too white and therefore underexposed. If the vessels in the lungs cannot be seen, the film is too black and therefore overexposed.

4. Rotation

The distance between each medial end of the clavicles and the interposed spinous process should be equal if there is no rotation.

5. Search pattern

Start at the center of the frontal film and work your way to the edges. As you do so, correlate with the lateral view. Look at the mediastinum, the lungs, the chest wall and lastly the diaphragm and upper abdomen. Look for any specific problems (see specific problems section).

B. Specific signs

1. Silhouette sign

If a water density process in the lung such as pneumonia is next to a water density structure such as the heart, the border between them is lost. This is called the *Silhouette sign.* Remember, there is no border between two same density structures in anatomical contact (The Basics; experiment 3).

The Silhouette sign helps to localize lesions in the lungs. For example, if an area of pneumonia obliterates the border between the lung and an anterior structure such as the heart, the pneumonia is located anteriorly (Fig.2-3). However, if the border between the lung and a posterior structure is obliterated, the pneumonia is located posteriorly in the chest.

The following is a list of commonly obliterated borders, and their associated lung lobes that lie in anatomic contact with them:

- Right heart border = right middle lobe pneumonia
- Left heart border = lingula (part of left upper lobe)
- Right hemidiaphragm = right lower lobe
- Left hemidiaphragm = left lower lobe
- Descending aorta = left lower lobe

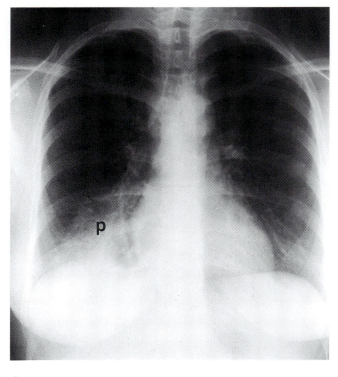

A

Fig.2-3: Silhouette sign. A. PA radiograph of the chest. A water density process (p, pneumonia) in the RLL obliterates the right hemidiaphragm. B. Lateral chest radiograph. The pneumonia is located in anterior segment of the RLL. C. PA chest radiograph. A pneumonia in the RML obliterates the right heart border. D. Lateral chest radiograph. The pneumonia is located in the RML.

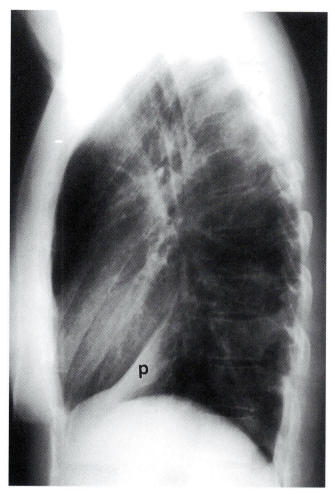

B

Fig.2-3 *(continued)*

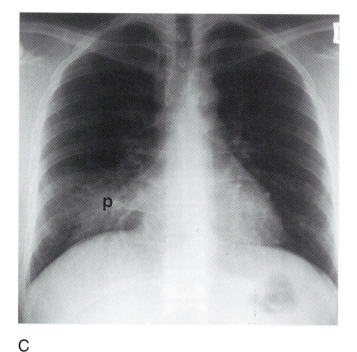

C

2. Air bronchogram sign

On the radiograph, the thin walls of bronchi are not visible because they are filled with air and are surrounded by air. If the surrounding alveoli, usually filled with air, become filled with a fluid density material, the air in the bronchi can be seen on the radiograph. The appearance of dark branching markings in abnormal white lung is called the *air bronchogram sign* (Fig.2-4). This sign is nonspecific as alveoli can be filled with pus, blood or fluid (pneumonia, hemorrhage or pulmonary edema respectively). Remember that if an air bronchogram is present, the lesion seen *must* be in the lung.

3. Kerly B sign (line)

Kerly B lines are small horizontal lines that are seen in the periphery of the lung. These lines are water density and *always* extend to the pleura (Fig.2-5). Kerly B lines are seen when there is increased fluid density material in the interlobular septa. This is often the result of pulmonary edema (e.g. *CHF-congestive heart failure*). Another cause to be considered is spread of tumor through the lymphatic system (*Lymphangitic carcinomatosis*).

D

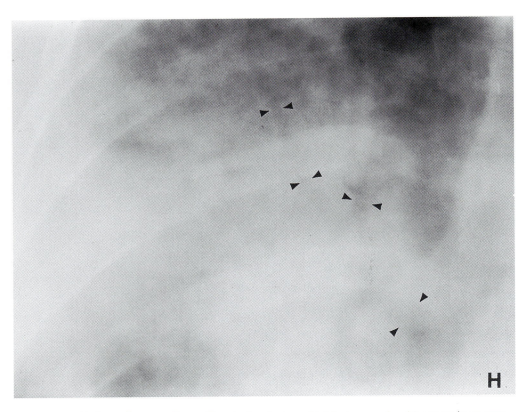

Fig.2-4: Air bronchogram sign.   The air density bronchi (black arrow heads) appear in an area of abnormally white lung. Heart (H).

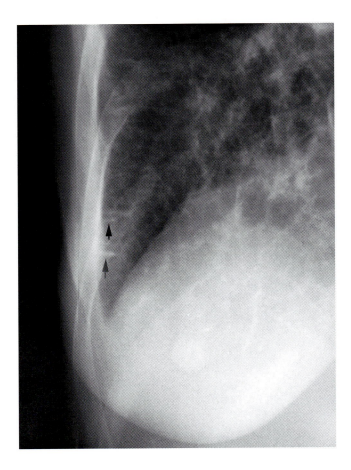

Fig.2-5: Kerly B sign. Small horizontal lines extend to the pleura (black arrow heads).

4. Snow ball sign

The *Snow ball sign* is used to determine whether a peripheral mass or nodule arises from the lung or from a surrounding structure. It is analogous to a snow ball thrown on a wall (Fig.2-6AC). If the nodule or mass looks like a snow ball just before impact, it is localized in the lung (Fig.2-6AB). However, if it looks like a flattened snow ball just after impact, it arises from a surrounding structure (chest wall, pleura or mediastium; Fig.2-6CD).

A

C

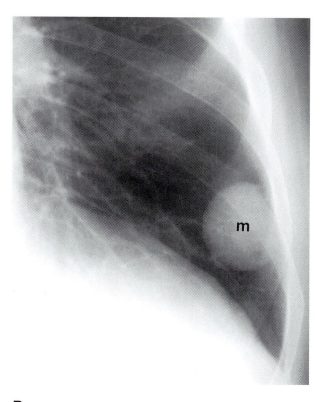

B

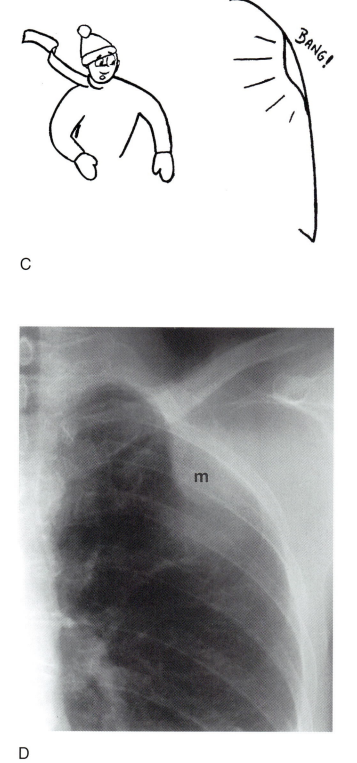

D

Fig.2-6:   Snow ball sign.   A. Drawing of a snow ball just before impact. B. PA chest radiograph. A mass (m) looks like a snow ball just before impact, and therefore is located in the lung. C. Drawing of a snow ball splattered about on a wall after impact. D A mass (m) looks like a flattened snow ball just after impact, and therefore is located in the chest wall or the pleura.

C. Lung disease patterns

1. Interstitial pattern

An interstitial pattern has the appearance of innumerable thin white lines randomly distributed in the lungs (Fig.2-7A). This pattern represents the presence of fluid density material in the interstitium (e.g. inflammatory fluid). Tiny white nodules are also occasionally seen. Interstitial patterns are otherwise known as *reticular pattern* and *reticulonodular pattern*.

2. Air space disease

An area of air space disease refers to a patch of white opacity, which results from the presence of fluid density material in the alveoli (e.g. pneumonia; Fig.2-7B). Air space disease is also called *consolidation*.

3. Honeycomb pattern

A Honeycomb pattern refers to an area of lung that takes on the appearance of a honeycomb (Fig.2-7C, 2-17). This pattern often signifies long standing interstitial lung disease and irreversible scarring (e.g. *fibrosing alveolitis, asbestosis*).

4. Miliary pattern

A miliary pattern refers to innumerable pellet size white dots appearing diffusely in both lungs (2-7D). This pattern is often seen in miliary tuberculosis.

III. Specific Problems

A. Mediastinum

1. Aortic laceration (wide mediastinum)

Aortic laceration occurs in significant trauma such as in a *Motor Vehicle Accident (MVA)*. Blood collects near the aortic arch. The mediastinal pleural and fat attempt to contain the hematoma, which becomes round and localized.

On the chest radiograph, the following findings are suggestive of aortic laceration and mediastinal hematoma (Fig.2-8):

1. the mediastinum may appear wide
2. the aortic arch becomes blurred
3. there may be blood over the apex of a lung appearing as a white crescent (*apical cap*)
4. the hematoma pushes the trachea to the right and the left main stem bronchus downward
5. the nasogastric tube, if present, may be pushed to the right

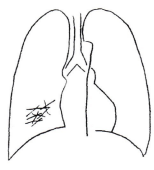

A

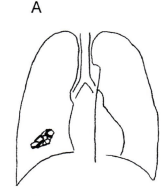

C

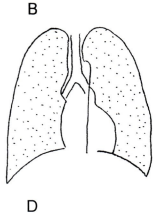

D

Fig.2-7: Lung disease patterns. A. An interstitial pattern is when there are innumerable thin white lines running in any direction in an area of the lung. B. Air space disease is a ill-defined white patch in a lung. C. A honeycomb pattern. D. A miliary pattern is innumerable pellet size white dots in both lungs.

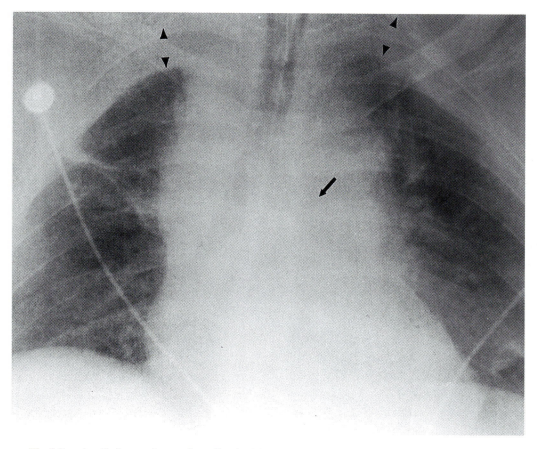

Fig.2-8: Aortic laceration and mediastinal hematoma. AP chest radiograph demonstrating a wide mediastinum, a blurred aortic arch, bilateral apical caps (black arrow heads), displaced left main stem bronchus downwards (black arrow).

Remember that the mediastinum is magnified on an AP view, and even more so, on a portable supine film. This may make it difficult to assess mediastinal widening.

2. Pneumomediastinum

Mediastinal air appears as black air density streaks on the radiograph (Fig.2-9). The air may outline mediastinal structures such as the aortic arch, and may even extend into the pericardial cavity (*pneumopericardium*).

Think about the thoracic structures that contain air. These include the lungs, trachea, and esophagus. Therefore, a lung laceration (*pneumothorax*), tracheal rupture, and esophageal rupture can all cause air in the mediastinum. Also, remember that the mediastinum is connected to the retroperitoneum, and that any cause of retroperitoneal air such as bowel perforation can track up into the mediastinum (discussed in Abdominal Radiograph chapter).

3. Enlarged cardiac silhouette

If the heart's largest transverse measurement is greater than half of the width of the chest, there is an enlarged cardiac silhouette.

The heart's silhouette may be enlarged because of the heart itself (*cardiomegaly*). This may occur because of congestive heart failure (*CHF*), incompetent cardiac valves or heart muscle disease (*cardiomyopathy*).

The "cardiac" silhouette is also enlarged when there is abnormal fluid in the pericardial cavity (*pericardial effusion*). The effusion and the heart itself are both fluid density and, therefore, cannot be differentiated on the chest radiograph.

B. Lungs/ pleura

1. Too white!

a. Pneumonia

Focal (air space disease) Pneumonia as a focal area of air space disease can cause a Silhouette or an Air Bronchogram sign (Fig.2-3). It may involve part or all of a lobe of the lung. This pattern is often caused by a bacterial infection.

Diffuse interstitial Diffuse interstitial pneumonia is primarily an infection of the interstitium of the lung. It is usually bilateral and often appears as multiple white lines. It is mainly caused by viruses and mycoplasma. Sometimes

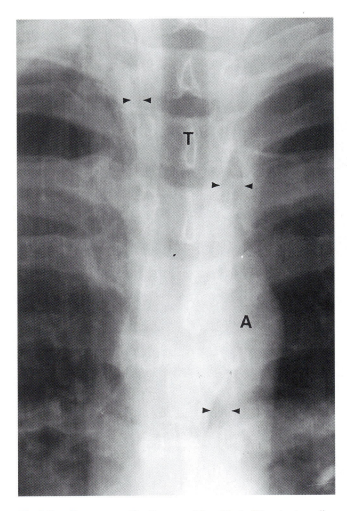

Fig.2-9: Pneumomediastinum. Magnified PA chest radiograph over the superior mediastinum demonstrating abnormal black streaks (black arrow heads) representing mediastinal air. Trachea (T). Aortic arch (A).

the infection cannot be contained in the interstitium and spills into the alveoli.

   Tuberculosis (TB), a special case TB is caused by inhalation of tiny droplets containing *Mycobacterium tuberculosis.* These bacteria are much like military soldiers parachuted into the lung. At first, the host's ground troops (the inflammatory cells) come to fight the intruders, which results in inflammation. This is called a *primary TB infection.* *M. tuberculosis* are more clever than average bacteria, and know better than to fight, so they go into hiding. This is called a *latent TB infection.* After weeks, months or sometimes even years, they come out of hiding. This is called a *secondary TB infection* or *reactivation TB.*

  Primary TB infection usually results in air space disease of one of the lower lobes, pleural effusions and hilar lymph node enlargement (Fig.2-10A). In latent TB infection, the

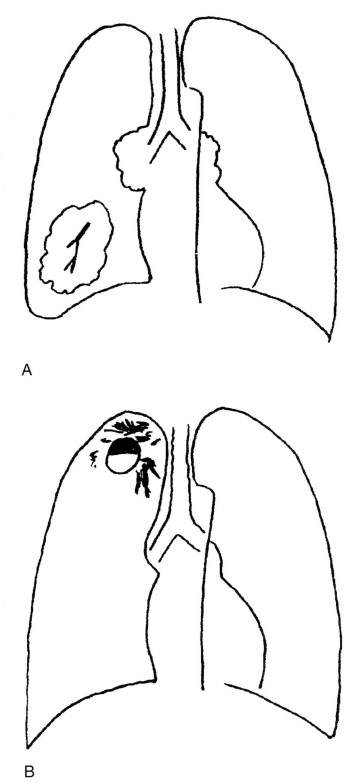

Fig.2-10: Tuberculosis (TB). A. Primary TB is characterized by air space disease in one of the lower lobes, pleural effusion and hilar lymph node enlargement. B. Secondary TB is characterized by upper lobe air space disease, which often progresses to scarring and cavity formation. C. PA chest radiograph demonstrating right upper lobe multiple cavities and scarring in a patient with secondary TB. Notice that disease has spread via the bronchi to the left lung (white arrow).

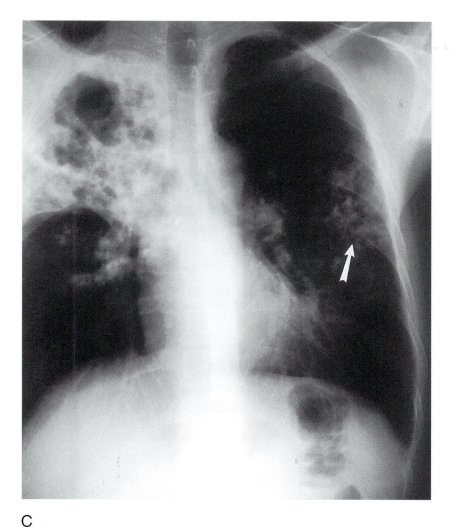

Fig. 2-10 (*continued*)

C

chest radiograph is often normal, although calcifications in the lungs or lymph nodes are occasionally seen. Secondary TB infection tends to occur in the upper lobes or in the superior aspects of the lower lobes. The involved lung often forms a cavity and scar tissue (Fig.2-10B, 2-10C).

Sometimes, the radiograph demonstrates very small white pellet-like nodules involving both lungs diffusely (Fig.2-11). This occurs in both primary and secondary infections and is called *miliary TB*. Remember that M. tuberculosis are like military soldiers. Take away the "t" in "military" to get the term *miliary*.

b. Atalectasis (collapse)

The innumerable alveoli that make up the lungs are analogous to air filled balloons. If for some reason air is resorbed from a significant portion of these structures, there will be loss of volume or collapse of the affected area (*atalectasis*). On the radiograph, the affected lung tissue is white (fluid density). This is not surprising since the alveoli no longer contain air. Sometimes, only a small number of alveoli are affected, which results in white streaks called "*plate-like atalectasis.*" However, collapse of an entire lobe or even an entire lung is frequently seen.

There are three main causes of atalectasis: obstruction, compression and traction. If a mass (e.g. tumor) or foreign body (e.g. peanut) causes obstruction of a bronchus, alveoli supplied by this bronchus will not fill with air and will collapse. Compression atalectasis, however, is due to any space occupying lesion that pushes against the alveoli and drives out the air. Examples of this form of collapse result from pneumothorax and pleural effusions. Lastly, traction atalectasis is due to scarring, which distorts the alveoli and contracts the lung. Such scarring may be caused by a severe infection, such as tuberculosis or chronic lung fibrosis.

Another important direct sign of collapse is the displacement of the interlobar fissure toward the collapsed lobe. When a portion of lung collapses and loses volume, it drags

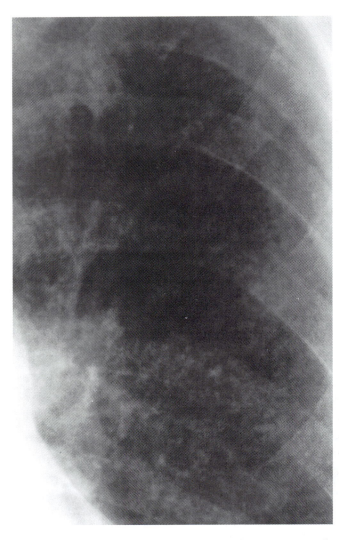

Fig.2-11: Miliary TB. Magnified view of a PA chest radiograph demonstrating small pellet-like nodules.

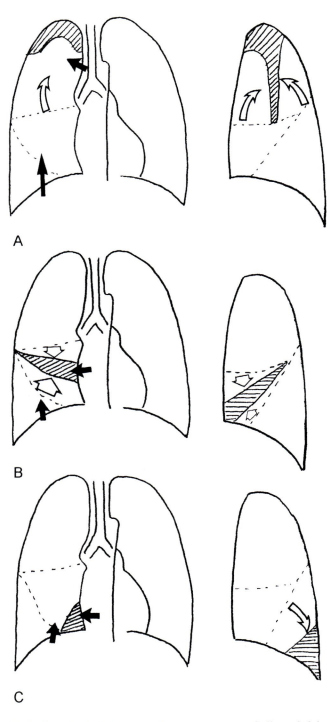

the adjacent fissure with it. Indirect signs are also often seen such as displacement of a diaphragm or mediastinal structures toward the area of volume loss. Collapse of each lobe has its own characteristic appearance on the chest radiograph (Fig.2-12, 2-13).

c. Cavity

A lung cavity appears as a thick white soft tissue density ring with a dark air density center. Often cavities are partially filled with fluid, giving rise to a straight horizontal line dividing the ring into a bottom white section and a top black section (air-fluid level; Fig.2-14). Cavities are often caused by abscesses, fugal pneumonia, granulomatous diseases such as TB, and tumors.

Fig.2-12: Typical lobar collapse patterns. Collapsed lobe (black lined area), displacement of fissures (open arrows), displacement of the mediastinum and hemidiaphragm (black arrows) is shown. A. Right upper lobe collapse. B. Right middle lobe collapse. C. Right lower lobe collapse. D. Left upper lobe collapse. E. Left lower lobe collapse.

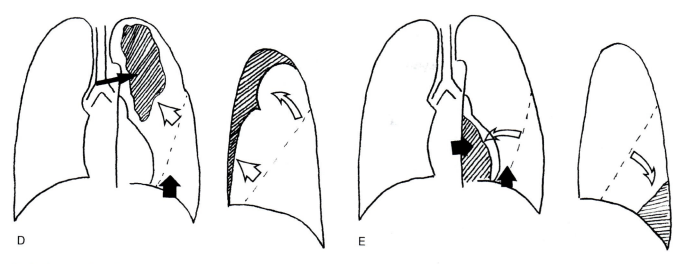

D E

Fig.2-12   (*continued*)

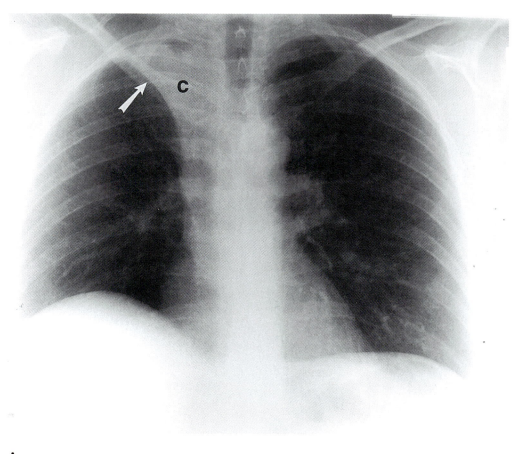

A

Fig.2-13:   Right upper lobe collapse.   A. PA chest radiograph B. Lateral chest radiograph. An abnormally white area is seen representing a collapsed right upper lobe (c). The right minor and major fissures are displaced superiorly (white arrows).

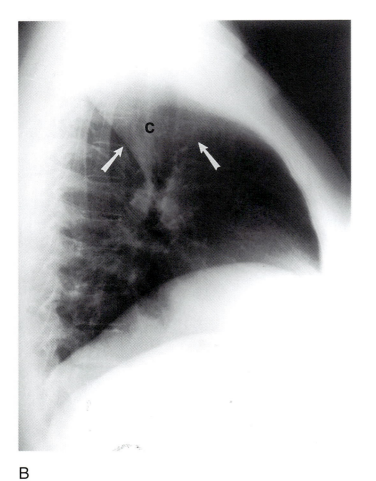

Fig.2-13   (*continued*)

B

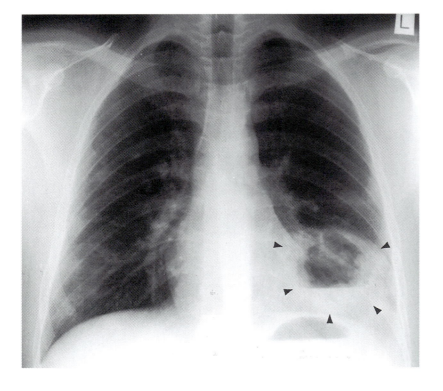

Fig.2-14:   Lung cavity (abscess).   PA chest radiograph demonstrating a left lower lobe cavity (black arrow heads). Notice the air fluid level in the cavity.

d. Pleural Effusion / Hemothorax / Empyema

A pleural effusion is simply a collection of fluid between the visceral pleura and the parietal pleura (i.e. *pleural space*). This fluid collection may be serous fluid (*pleural effusion*), blood (*hemothorax*), or pus (*empyema*). In the case of empyema, there may be small bubbles of air in the pus.

On an upright PA film, fluid collects in the lateral costophrenic angle due to gravity, giving it a blunted appearance (Fig.2-15A). The posterior costophrenic angle is the deepest, and fluid collects there first. This angle is hidden by the dome of the diaphragm on a PA view. However, it is well seen on the lateral view (Fig.2-15B). For this reason, the upright lateral view is superior to the PA for demonstrating small amounts of pleural fluid.

When patients are too sick to have an upright PA view of the chest, then an AP supine view is taken. Recall that patients in this view are lying on their back. If an effusion is present, it will layer between the posterior chest wall and the lung due to gravity. On the AP view, the affected hemi-thorax will therefore be diffusely increased in density (whiter than the normal side).

When in doubt, order a decubitus view with the patient lying down on the side of the suspected effusion. This will bring the fluid between the lung and the chest wall where it is easy to see (Fig.2-15C).

Sometimes the parietal and visceral pleura are stuck to each other (*adhesion*). In this situation, a pleural effusion may not be able to move when the patient changes position. The fluid may even be stuck in one of the fissures mimicking the appearance of a lung mass (pseudo-tumor). Immobile pleural fluid is called a *loculated effusion*.

e. Congestive heart failure (CHF)

CHF occurs when the heart becomes unable to pump out the same amount of blood that it is receiving. The heart becomes enlarged (*cardiomegaly*). When there is left ventricular failure, fluid backs up in the pulmonary veins and lung. Fluid seeps out into the interstitium first and then eventually into the alveoli and pleural space.

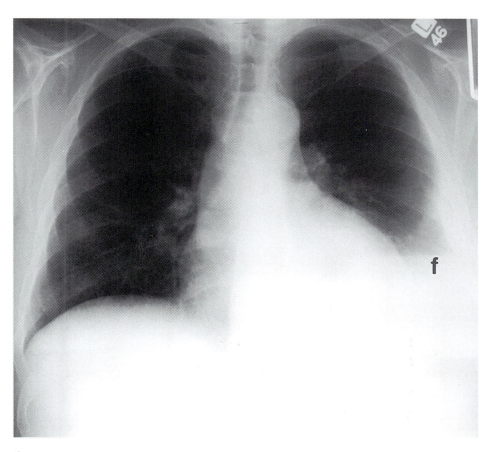

Fig.2-15: Left pleural effusion. A. PA chest radiograph demonstrating fluid (f) in the left costophrenic angle. B. Lateral chest radiograph demonstrating fluid around the left lower lobe and in the left oblique fissure (black arrow heads). C. Left lateral decubitus view of the chest demonstrating fluid between the chest wall and the left lung (black arrow heads).

A

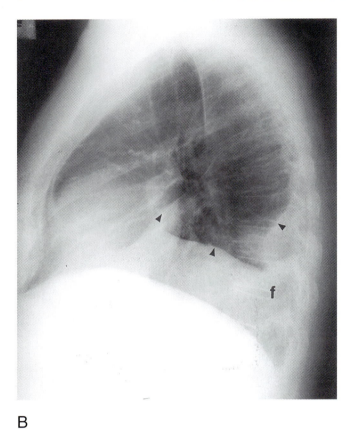

B

On the radiograph, look for the following findings (Fig.2-16A, 2-16B):

1. *Vascular redistribution:* blood vessels in the upper lung zones become larger than the ones in lower lung zones (the inverse of normal)

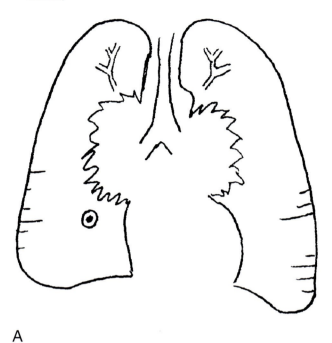

A

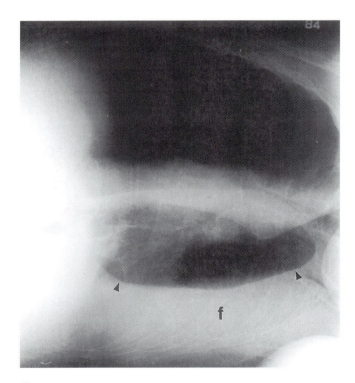

C

Fig.2-15 (*continued*)

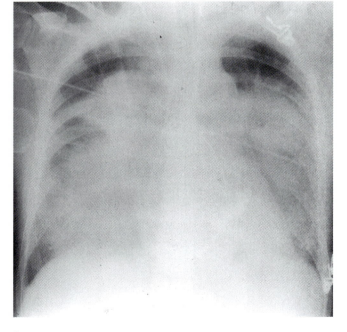

B

Fig.2-16: Congestive heart failure (CHF).   A. Common findings in CHF on a chest radiograph are vascular redistribution, Kerly B lines, peribronchial cuffing, pleural effusions and a batwing distribution of air space disease. B. PA chest radiograph demonstrating a typical batwing distribution of air space disease.

2. *Interstitial pattern* and *Kerly B lines*
3. *Peribrochial cuffing:* bronchi seen head on are surrounded by fluid
4. *Pleural effusions*
5. *Batwing pattern* (symmetrical air space disease in the lung adjacent to the hila)

f. Chronic interstitial lung disease

A discussion of chronic lung diseases is beyond the scope of this book. Remember that if an abnormal white area has not changed compared to a remote previous exam, there is likely chronic lung disease. Also, remember that the honey comb pattern previously discussed is suggestive of scarring (Fig.2-17).

g. Nodule/Mass

Nodules and masses in the lung appear as round white fluid density lesions (Fig.2-6A, 2-6B). If the lesion measures less than 3 cm, it is called a nodule. If it is larger than 3 cm, it is called a mass.

A nodule/mass is caused by either a malignant (e.g. lung cancer, metastasis) or benign process (e.g. *hamartoma, granuloma*). Primary lung cancers tend to have ill-defined, spiculated borders, and grow over time. Metastases tend to produce multiple smooth round lung nodules, often of variable size. Benign lesions tend to be small, well defined, smooth, round and maybe calcified. They usually are stable in size when compared to prior films.

2. Too black!

a. Pneumothorax / Tension pneumothorax

Pneumothorax is air between the parietal pleura and the visceral pleura, usually arising from a lung injury. Remember that air has a tendency to rise to the highest point in the chest (contrary to fluid).

In an upright PA film, look for a black crescent over the apex of the lung. In addition, the visceral pleura is often seen as a thin white line under the black crescent, since it is flanked by air on each side (Fig.2-18A). One should not be able to see branching white blood vessels peripheral to this line. Taking a film during expiration often makes a pneumothorax more visible, because the amount of pleural air remains the same although the lungs become smaller.

On a supine AP, the air rises to the anterior and lateral costophrenic angles (sulci). This is no surprise since they are the highest region in the pleural cavity when the patient is lying down. This makes the lateral sulcus look abnormally dark and deep (i.e. deep sulcus sign).

In the case of *tension pneumothorax,* a lung injury causing leakage of air into the pleural space may form a one-way valve. This valve lets air escape into the pleural cavity during inspiration only. With every breath the patient takes, more air seeps into the pleural cavity, and becomes trapped. Eventually, the air pushes the medi-

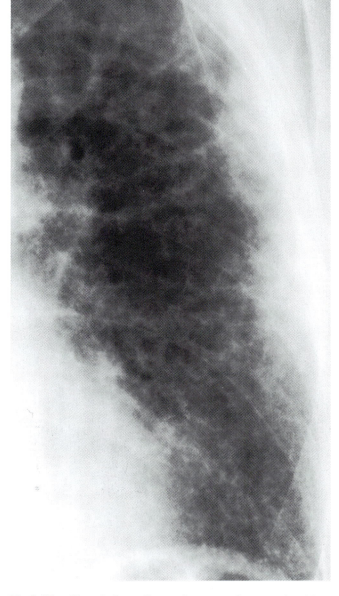

Fig.2-17: Chronic lung disease (honeycomb pattern). Magnified view of a PA chest radiograph demonstrating an honeycomb pattern representing lung scarring.

astinum and the diaphragm, and the heart becomes unable to pump blood because of the tension inside the chest. This is obviously an emergency, which requires immediate pressure relief (e.g. large bore needle or chest tube insertion; Fig.2-18B).

b. Emphysema

Emphysema is caused by chronic airway obstruction resulting in destruction of alveoli. Lungs contain more air than

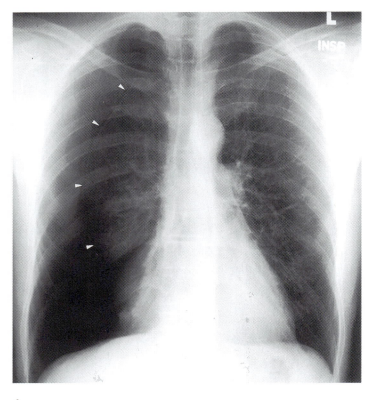

A

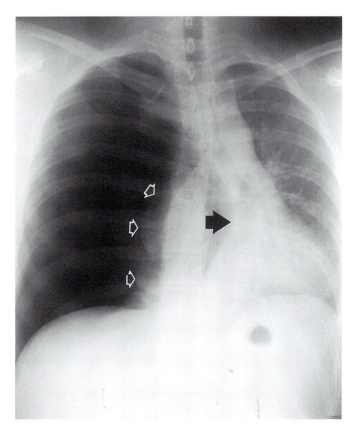

B

Fig.2-18: Pneumothorax and tension pneumothorax. A. Magnified view of a PA chest radiograph of a right pneumothorax. The visceral pleura (arrow heads) is seen as a thin white line. B. PA chest radiograph demonstrating an abnormally black right hemithorax. The right lung (white open arrows) has been pushed medially. The mediastinum is shifted to the left (black arrow). This appearance is typical of tension pneumothorax.

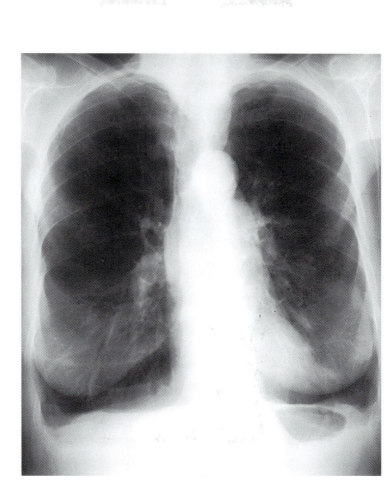

A

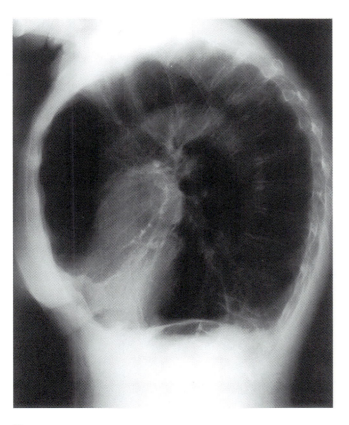

B

Fig.2-19: Emphysema. A. PA chest radiograph demonstrating lungs that are too black, decreased number of vessels, curved course of vessels and flattened hemi-diaphragms. B. Lateral view of the chest demonstrating flattened hemidiaphragms and barrel chest deformity.

normal because the airway obstruction causes air trapping. Sometimes, ball-shaped collections of air develop, which are called bullae.

On the radiograph, there is an overall decrease in lung density (too black). This makes sense since the fluid density alveolar walls are being destroyed and air is trapped in the lungs. Also, because of tissue destruction, there are fewer visible blood vessels. Ones that are seen sometimes take an abnormal curved course because they are going around destroyed lung. Lastly, there is flattening of the diaphragm because of hyperinflation of the lungs (Fig. 2-19A, 2-19B).

c. Pulmonary embolism

Pulmonary embolism occurs when a clot (e.g. from a leg vein) is dislodged. The clot then travels to the lungs and blocks a pulmonary artery. This prevents the blood from getting to the area of lung supplied by the affected vessel where it would get oxygenated.

The chest radiograph often is close to normal with pulmonary embolism. Sometimes a focal, black, wedge-shaped area is seen, as blood does not fill the blood vessels after the embolism. Nonspecific signs include atelectasis and pleural effusion. Occasionally, a white wedge-shaped area of air space disease is seen due to post-obstruction infarction (*Hampton's hump*).

C. Chest wall

1. Rib fracture

Fractures often occur at the lateral aspect of the rib where it is curved the most, and therefore the weakest. If rib fractures are seen, look for a pneumothorax! The jagged fracture edges sometimes puncture the lung. Although painful, rib fractures alone are not of any major clinical consequence.

2. Subcutaneous emphysema

Subcutaneous emphysema refers to air under the skin, either in the chest wall or in the neck. This is observed on the radiograph as dark air density streaks in the soft tissue.

Think about structures that normally contain air such as the lungs, the esophagus, and the trachea. There is also air surrounding the patient's skin. The source of subcutaneous air can therefore be a lung laceration (pneumothorax), esophageal rupture, tracheal laceration, or skin laceration. Mediastinal air can also extend to the neck and chest wall.

D. Diaphragm

1. Rupture

Diaphragmatic rupture is caused by significant trauma and occurs on the left side 9 times out of 10. Abdominal structures such as the stomach, the spleen or the large bowel may herniate through the tear.

On the radiograph, the affected diaphragm appears elevated. There may be an air fluid level, implying the presence of the bowel in the chest. The nasogastric tube tip, if present, may be in the chest. Also, look for displacement of the mediastinum away from the tear. This occurs because of structures herniated to the chest, which take up space and push the mediastinum away (Fig.2-20).

2. Hiatus hernia

A hiatus hernia is slippage of the top part of the stomach (*fundus*) into the mediastinum through the esophageal hiatus of the diaphragm. This is a common and relatively benign condition. On the radiograph, the gastric fundus may appear as a fluid density mass, or an air fluid level behind the heart in the mediastinum (Fig.2-21A, 2-21B).

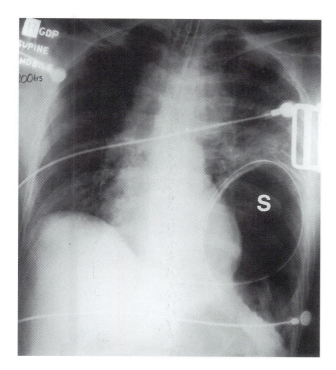

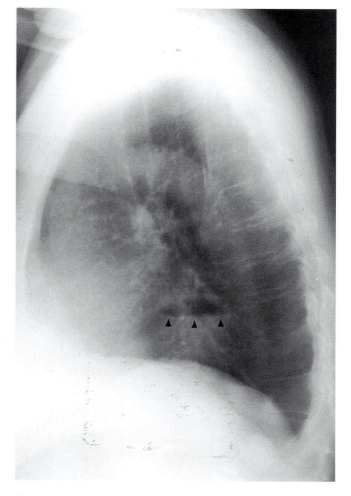

Fig.2-20: Left diaphragmatic rupture. PA chest radiograph showing that the stomach (S) has herniated into the left hemithorax through a defect in the diaphragm. The nasogastric tube is seen in the stomach. Notice also that the mediastinum is pushed to the right.

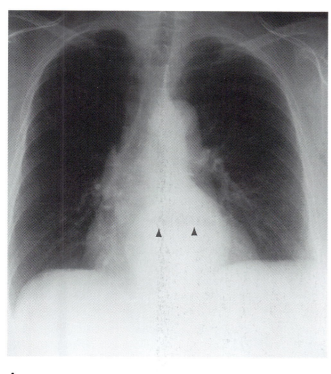

A

Fig.2-21: Hiatus hernia. A. PA chest radiograph showing air fluid level of the stomach, which herniated through the diaphragm. B. Lateral chest radiograph.

B

Chapter 3.   Abdominal Radiograph

I. Radiographic anatomy

The three most commonly used views of the abdomen are *supine* (lying on the back), *erect* (standing up) and *left lateral decubitus* (left side down) views. The abdomen is divided into 4 quadrants: the right upper quadrant (RUQ), left upper quadrant (LUQ), right lower quadrant (RLQ) and the left lower quadrant (LLQ). In the LUQ, the gastric bubble is often seen. The remainder of bowel contains variable amounts of gas. Only the inner aspect of bowel that contains air can be visualized. The outer limits of the bowel wall are impossible to see. This is because bowel is of fluid density. Gasless loops adjacent to each other are all of the same fluid density and, therefore, their contour will not be seen.

From most proximal to distal, the small bowel is composed of the duodenum, the jejunum and the ileum, which usually contain less gas than the large bowel. It is located in the middle of the abdomen and has folds, having the density of fluid, crossing the entire width of the bowel (*valvulae coniventes*). The large bowel (the *colon*) is composed of the appendix, the cecum, the ascending colon, hepatic flexure, transverse colon, splenic flexure, descending colon, sigmoid colon and rectum. Large bowel is located peripherally in the abdomen and therefore looks like a picture frame (Fig.3-1A). It contains folds that do not cross the entire length of the bowel width, called *haustra*.

Remember that there are bilateral *flank fat stripes* adjacent to the ascending and descending colon. The distance between a flank stripe and adjacent colon should not be greater than the width of a pinky finger.

The abdomen is divided into two cavities. The *peritoneal cavity* is lined by a thin layer of tissue (*peritoneum*) that wraps around most of the bowel, the spleen and most of the liver. The peritoneum forms a recess lateral to both the ascending and descending colon (*paracolic gutters*). The *retroperitoneal cavity* is located behind the peritoneal cavity. It contains the pancreas, kidneys, psoas muscles, aorta, bladder, ascending and descending colon and the rectum. On the radiograph, the contour of several organs are seen (Fig.3-1B).

The mesenteric arteries (not seen on film) arise from the aorta to supply blood to bowel. The blood is then brought to the liver from the bowel via the *portal vein*. After being filtered, the blood exits the liver into the inferior vena cava to join the general circulation. In addition to filtering blood, the liver makes a fluid called *bile,* which is important in digestion. This digestive juice gets to the duodenum via a system of tubes called the *biliary system*. Notice that the liver is of homogeneous fluid density, and that portal vein and bile duct are not normally seen. This is because the liver, blood and bile are all of the same fluid density.

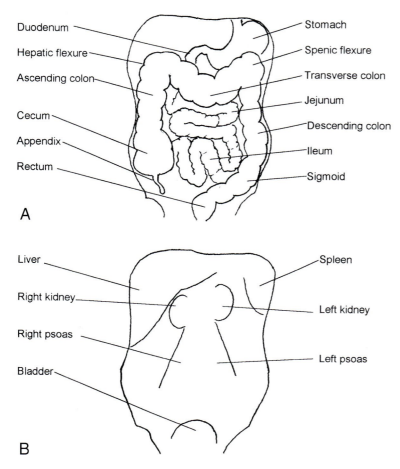

A

B

Fig.3-1: Abdominal anatomy. A. Gastrointestinal anatomy. B. Abdominal radiographic shadows.

II. Approach

Plain abdominal radiographs are a lot like champagne: one can tell a lot by looking at the gas bubbles. Use the following mnemonic to approach this exam systematically. Mnemonic: **Free ABDO**

Free Free fluid:

Look at the distance between the lateral fat stripes and the adjacent segment of colon and for pooling of the bowel to the center of the supine film (discussed in free fluid section).

A Air:

1. Air outside the bowel lumen

Look for any evidence of free intraperitoneal air, retroperitoneal air, branching air in the liver, and abcesses. Look also for evidence of air in the bowel wall.

2. Air inside the bowel lumen

Look for any dilated bowel and air fluid levels.

B Bowel wall thickening:

Look for specific signs of bowel wall thickening.

D Densities:

Look at the bony structures for any gross abnormalities (discussed in bone radiology chapters). Look for any abnormal calcifications such as appendicolith, gallbladder and renal stones, pancreatic and aortic calcifications.

O Organs:

Look at the outline of the liver, the spleen, the kidneys, and the bladder for any enlargement, abnormality or loss of contour.

III. Specific problems

A. Free fluid

Free fluid in the peritoneal cavity (*ascites*) and blood are the same density on the radiograph and therefore cannot be differentiated. Look at the distance between the colon and the flank fat stripe. If this distance is greater than the width of a pinky finger, there is likely free peritoneal fluid in the paracolic gutters. (Fig.3-2).

When large amounts of free fluid are present, there may be a diffuse increased opacification (too white) in the abdomen on the supine film. As air rises much like in hot air balloons, the bowel floats to the center of the anterior abdominal wall, which is the highest point in the abdomen. Therefore, the bowel tends to collect in the center of the abdomen.

B. Air out of bowel lumen

1. Intraperitoneal air (free air)

Normally, there is no air outside of the bowel in the peritoneal cavity. Intraperitoneal free air signifies that the bowel may be perforated. This is a catastrophic event requiring ur-

gent surgery, because bowel contents seep into the sterile peritoneal cavity and cause infection. Frequent locations of bowel perforation are the duodenum secondary to *peptic ulcer disease,* and the colon secondary to *diverticulitis, colon cancer* or *obstruction.*

Look for air under the diaphragm on the upright abdominal view or chest radiograph. Free air is easiest to see on the right side because it becomes interposed between the liver and the diaphragm, which are two fluid density structures (Fig.3-3A). On the left side, the stomach may contain air, making the interpretation of the film more difficult. Remember that in some patients, large bowel is interposed between the liver and the diaphragm, which may lead to incorrect diagnosis of free intraperitoneal air (*Chilaiditi's syndrome*).

On the left lateral decubitus view, free air collects under the patient's right lateral flank (Fig.3-3B). In women, the free

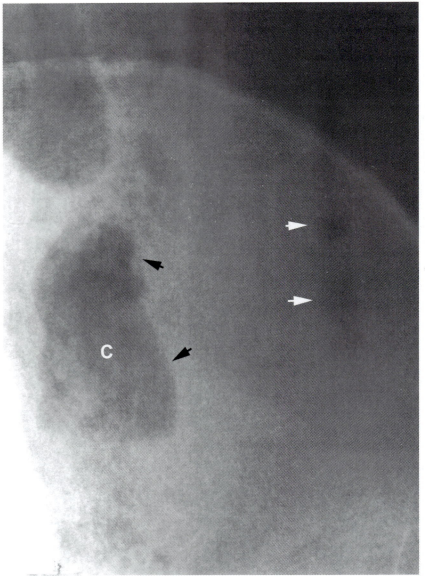

Fig.3-2: Free fluid (ascites). Magnified abdominal radiograph of the left lower quadrant. Free fluid separates the lateral wall (black arrows) of the descending colon (C) from the left flank stripe (vertical dark band shown by white arrows). Distance between the wall and the stripe should be no greater than the width of a small finger.

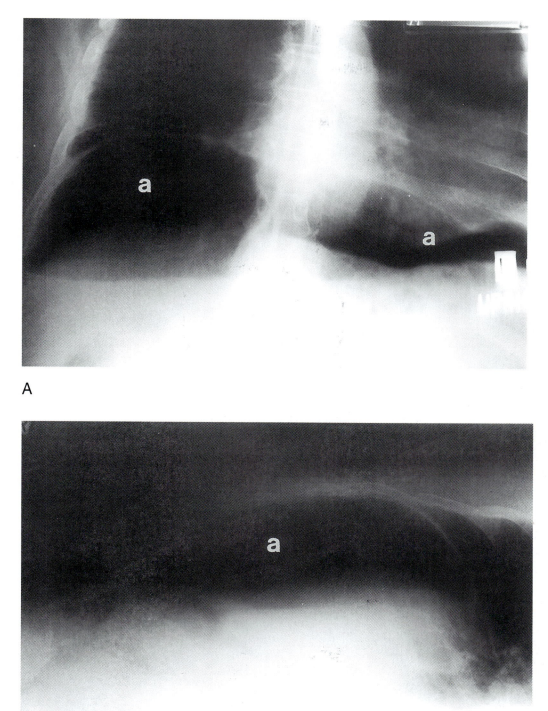

A

B

Fig.3-3:   Free intraperitoneal air (a).   A. Upright abdominal radiograph demonstrating free in-traperitoneal air (a) between the diaphragm and the liver. B. Left lateral decubitus view of the ab-domen showing air between the liver and the patient's right flank. C. Rigler's sign. Both sides of the bowel wall (black arrow heads) can be seen because it is outlined by free intraperitoneal air and air inside the bowel.

air may be seen adjacent to the right iliac bone because of a wider configuration of the hips.

Remember that bowel is only seen on the radiograph when it contains air, which outlines the inside of the bowel wall. Bowel that does not contain air is of fluid density and blends with other fluid density structures around it (other bowel loops), which makes it invisible on the radiograph. When there is free air, the normally invisible outer aspect of the bowel can be seen; air inside and outside the bowel enables one to see both the outer and inner aspects of the bowel. This finding, called *Rigler's sign,* is most frequently seen on a supine view of the abdomen and implies free abdominal air (Fig.3-3C).

Remember that free air is a normal finding after abdominal surgery, because air is introduced into the peritoneal cavity during the operation. On average, it takes about 10 days for this intraperitoneal air to be resorbed. More importantly, the amount of free air should always decrease on subsequent radiographs. A sudden increase in the amount of the free abdominal air implies bowel perforation.

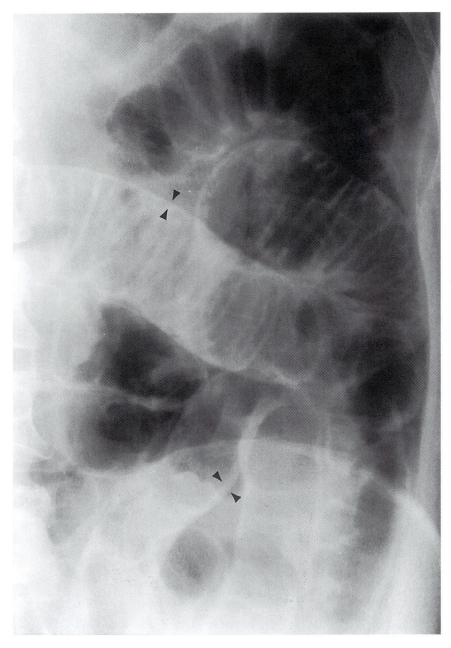

Fig.3-3 (*continued*)

C

2. Retroperitoneal air

Parts of the duodenum, and the ascending, descending and sigmoid colon are retroperitoneal structures. Therefore if they perforate, air may seep out into the retoperitoneal space.

On the radiograph, air may outline retroperitoneal structures such as the kidneys and the iliopsoas muscle, making their margins more visible. Abnormal air streaks extending into the iliopsoas muscle may also be seen.

3. Branching air in the liver

The liver is normally of homogeneous fluid density. The presence of branching darker areas within the liver is abnor-mal and suggests that there is either air in the biliary tree (*pneumobilia*) or in the portal venous system.

a. Pneumobilia

Air in the biliary tree most often is the result of bile duct manipulation (i.e. *sphincterotomy*). It may also signify dangerous pathology such as *emphysematous cholecystitis* (gas producing gallbladder infection; Fig.3-4). Because bile flows towards the hilum of the liver, pneumobilia often has the appearance of dark branching structures near the hilum of the liver (Fig.3-5A).

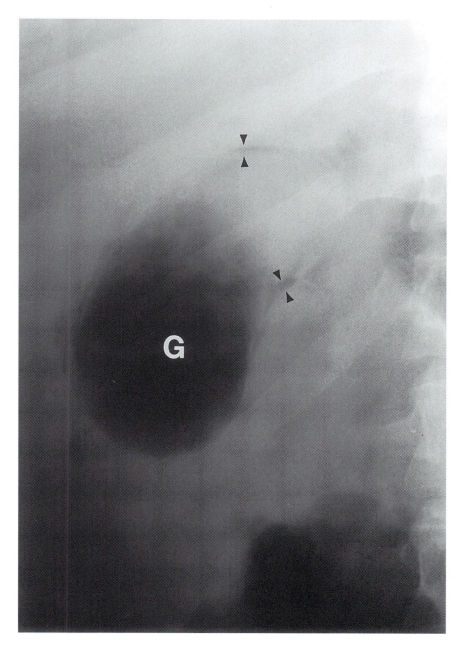

Fig.3-4: Emphysematous cholycystitis. Magnified view showing an air filled gall-bladder (G). There is also air in the wall of the gallbladder (black arrow heads).

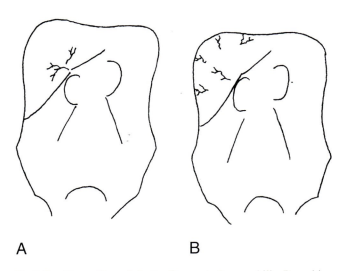

A   B

Fig.3-5:   Branching air in the liver   A. Pneumobilia. Branching black air near the hilum of the liver. B. Portal venous air. Branching black air throughout the liver including the periphery.

b. Portal venous air

Portal vein gas signifies that there has been a devastating event in the abdomen such as a massive bowel infarction. Since portal venous flow is from the hilum to the periphery of the liver, portal venous gas often appears as dark branching structures throughout the liver, including the periphery (Fig.3-5B).

4. Abscess

An abscess often appears on the radiograph as a black air collection, often in an area that does not correlate with the normal location of bowel. It does not have normal bowel features such as haustrations (large bowel) or valvulae coniventes (small bowel). Furthermore, an abscess usually remains at the same location, whereas air moves within the bowel on sequential films.

5. Pneumatosis (air in the bowel wall)

Air in the bowel wall may indicate impending bowel perforation or gangrene. It may also signify that the bowel is not receiving adequate blood supply (*bowel ischemia or infarct*). Pneumatosis appears as linear black streaks in bowel wall (fig.3-6).

C. Air in the bowel lumen (dilated bowel)

Bowel contains a variable amount of air. Don't worry if a large amount of gas is present, as long as the bowel is not dilated. As discussed in the anatomy section, small and large bowel are distinguished both by location and by the type of folds displayed. For each bowel segment , a critical bowel diameter can be used to indicate dilation.

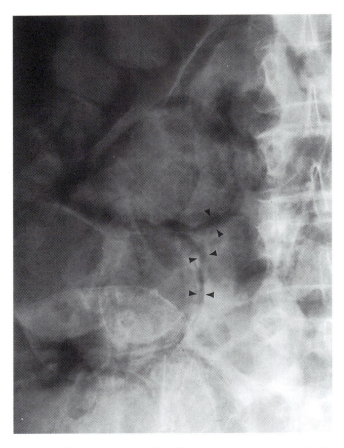

Fig.3-6:   Pneumatosis.   Magnified view showing air within the bowel wall (black arrow heads).

On the radiograph, look for bowel diameter greater than:

- 3 cm for the small bowel
- 6 cm for the large bowel (except cecum)
- 9 cm for the cecum

Remember that a straight horizontal line with air above and fluid below is called an *air-fluid level* and, is a finding that *must* be explained. Air fluid levels are seen on both erect and decubitus films.

1. Ileus

Ileus means that loops of bowel become paralyzed. In this situation, bowel dilates because of gas collection. Ileus can be localized (e.g. near an inflammatory process) or generalized (e.g. secondary to certain drugs, surgery or pain). Look at the erect film for air fluid levels.

2. Bowel obstruction

Bowel obstruction is caused by several problems, such as bowel cancer or adhesions. The bowel proximal to the obstruction dilates and more distal bowel collapses. Therefore, if there is only small bowel dilatation, the location of the obstruction is in the small bowel (Fig.3-7A, 3-7B). However, if the colon is dilated (with or without small bowel dilatation), large bowel obstruction may be suspected (Fig.3-8A, 3-8B).

Determine if the obstruction is *complete* or *partial*. This is clinically important since completely obstructed patients require an operation. Look at the distal bowel such as the rectum to see if it contains air. If it does, there is air seeping past the obstruction (i.e. partial). However, if there is no air in distal bowel such as the rectum, the obstruction is complete. Look at the erect film for air fluid levels.

3. Volvulus

Volvulus occurs when the bowel twists on itself, thereby causing obstruction. The most common type is volvulus of the sigmoid.

a. Sigmoid volvulus

Twisted sigmoid often appears on the radiograph as a dilated loop of large bowel in the lower abdomen, resembling a *coffee bean* or an *inverted U* (Fig.3-9A). The remainder of the colon is usually dilated.

b. Cecal volvulus

When twisted, the cecum leaves the right lower quadrant to look like a second stomach bubble in the middle of the abdomen (Fig.3-9B). There is often associated small bowel dilatation with cecal volvulus.

D. Bowel wall thickening

The bowel wall may thicken in inflammatory bowel diseases or bowel ischemia. In such cases, the loops of bowel

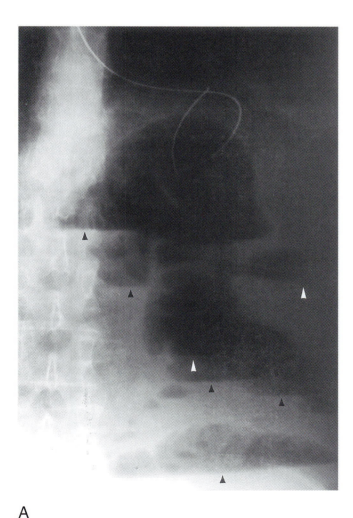

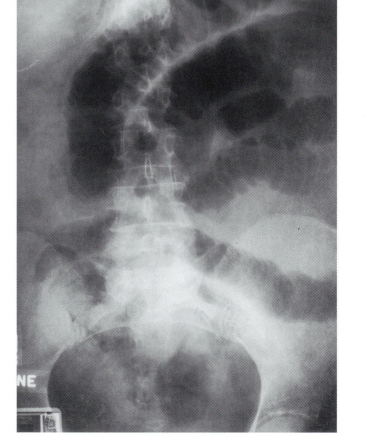

A

B

Fig.3-7: Small bowel obstruction. A. Upright abdominal radiograph. Small bowel dilatation with multiple fluid levels (arrow heads) is seen without air in the large bowel. B. Supine abdominal radiograph showing dilatation of small bowel.

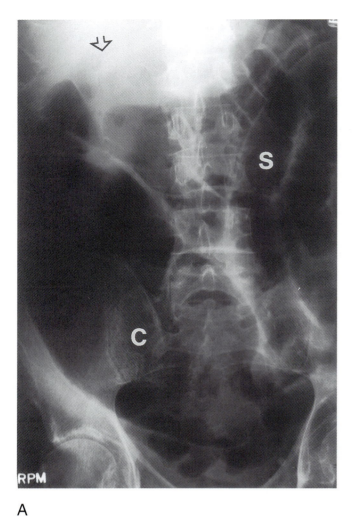

A

Fig.3-8: Large bowel obstruction. A. Supine abdominal radiograph showing dilation of the ascending colon (C) and the small bowel (S). The point of obstruction (open arrow) is seen at the hepatic flexure. B. Left lateral decubitus also showing several air fluid levels (arrow heads).

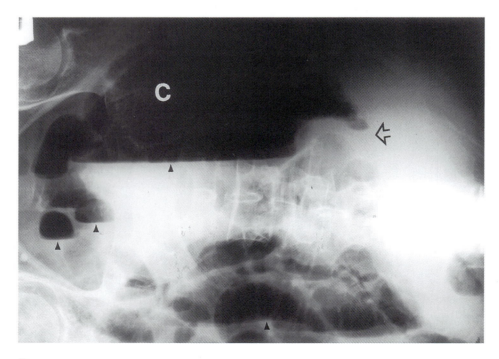

B

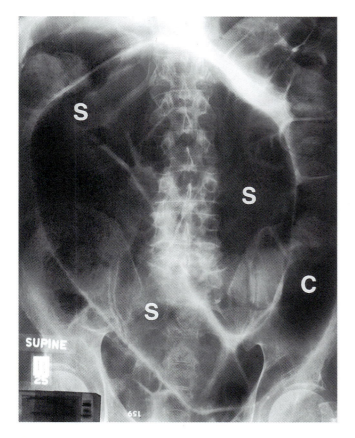

A

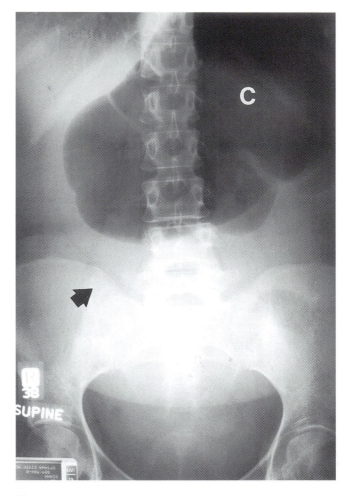

B

Fig.3-9: Bowel volvulus. A. Sigmoid volvulus. Abdominal radiograph showing a twisted and dilated sigmoid colon (S) taking on the appearance of a "coffee bean". Dilated descending colon (C). B. Cecal volvulus. Abdominal radiograph showing a dilated cecum (C) in the left upper part of the abdomen. A black arrow shows the direction of the abnormal displacement of the cecum.

demonstrate narrowing of the lumen and thickening of folds. In the large bowel, the wall may look like it has been indented by someone's thumb (*thumb printing*). Because the abnormal bowel walls are thickened, one often sees apparently increased distance between bowel loops or *loop separation.*

E. Densities (white)

1. Bones

Look at the bony structures of the vertebral column and pelvis for any gross abnormality (discussed in the bone radiology chapters).

2. Appendicolith

Although appendicitis is a clinical diagnosis, in about 10% of patients a small calcification is seen in the RLQ (ap-

pendicolith). There may also be focal small bowel ileus at this location.

3. Stones

Sometimes in the RUQ, gallbladder stones can be seen (Fig.3-10). Their appearance varies from that of one distinct stone to several small stones. These move when the patient changes position, as the gallbladder itself is mobile. Renal and ureteric stones are also sometimes visible (discussed in the Intravenous Pyelogram (IVP) chapter).

4. Pancreatic calcifications

Several small white calcifications may be seen across the midline in the area of the pancreas. This appearance is associated with *chronic pancreatitis.*

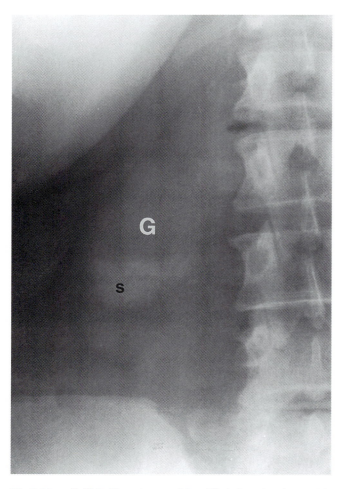

Fig.3-10: Gallbladder stones. Magnified view showing multiple small stones (s) in the gallbladder (G).

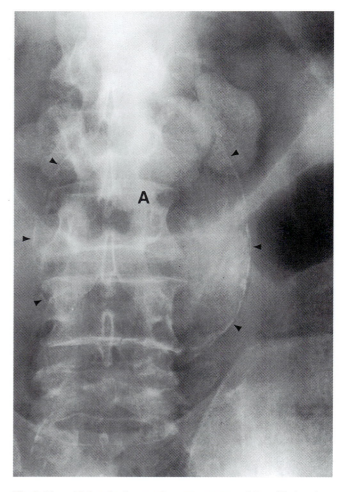

Fig.3-11: Abdominal aortic aneurysm. Magnified view showing the calcified wall (arrow heads) of an abdominal aortic aneurysm (A).

5. Abdominal aortic aneurysm (AAA)

In artherosclerosis of the aorta, bilateral curvilinear calcifications can sometimes be seen adjacent to the lumbar spine. If distance between these calcifications is greater than 3 cm, there is an abdominal aortic aneurysm (Fig.3-11). This condition places the patient at increased risk of abdominal aortic rupture and bleeding in the retroperitoneal cavity.

F. Organs

Most solid organs are surrounded by fat in the abdomen. This allows visualization of their outline. The liver and spleen may have an enlarged contour (*hepatosplenomegaly*). The kidney shadows may also be enlarged, missing, or display an abnormal mass (Discussed in IVP chapter).

Chapter 4.   Intravenous Pyelogram (IVP)

I. Radiographic anatomy

An IVP is analogous to two kids blowing through a straw into a balloon. They first take a deep breath. As they blow, their faces become blushed and the balloon enlarges (Fig.4-1A).

The IVP is a series of abdominal films taken sequentially over time. The first image is a plain radiograph of the abdomen (*Scout film*). On this image, one should see the kidney and bladder contours. The kidneys on the scout are analogous the kids' faces and the bladder is analogous to the balloon. The two kidneys are normally 3 to 4 lumbar vertebrae in length. The right kidney is lower then the left one because it is pushed down by the liver.

The other films are taken after IV contrast injection. As the kidneys filter blood and excrete urine, the urinary system becomes outlined by the white contrast material. This is analogous to the air flow going through the straw. One should see the whitened kidneys (*nephrograms*), which are analogous to the blushed faces of the boys in our story. The collecting systems, composed of the calyces, the infundibulae, the renal pelvices, are analogous to the kids' cheeks. In addition, one can visualize the ureteropelvic junctions (UPJ), the ureters, and the ureterovesicular junctions (UVJ), which represent the straws (Fig.4-2). The whitened bladder is analogous to the inflated balloon.

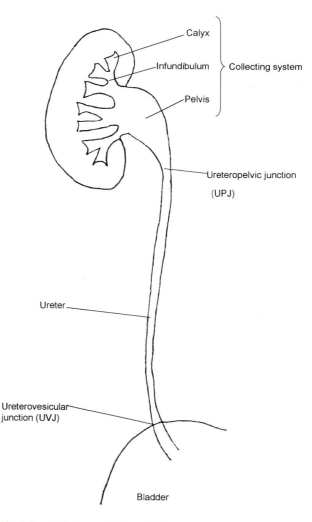

Fig.4-2:   **Urinary system anatomy.**

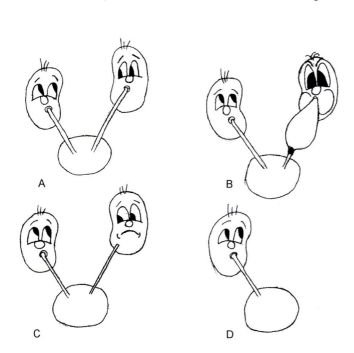

Fig.4-1:   The kids.   A. Two kids blowing through a straw in a balloon is analogous to the urinary system. B. Pebble obstructing a straw is analogous to a stone obstructing a ureter. C. One kid not blowing into a straw is analogous to a non-functioning kidney. D. An absent kid is analogous to an absent kidney.

II. Approach

A. Scout film

Approach the scout film as an abdominal radiograph (see Abdominal Radiograph chapter). Pay particular attention to the urinary system.

Look for:

1. *Kidney and bladder contours* (size and shape)
2. *Kidney stones* (white calcification over a kidney shadow)
3. *Ureteric stone* (white calcification along the course of the ureters)

B. Contrast injected films

Contrast films are usually taken at 1, 5 and 15 minutes after injection. Compare one side to the other. Look at:

1. *Nephrograms*
   • Absent: The kidney on contrast injection film does not whiten compared to the scout film.

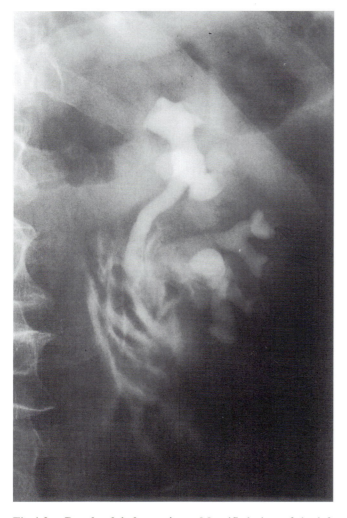

Fig.4-3: Renal pelvis laceration. Magnified view of the left kidney after contrast injection showing white streaks, which represent contrast leaking out of the renal pelvis into surrounding tissues.

   • Delayed: The kidney is not whiter on the 5 minute film than on the scout.
   • Hyperdense: Too white
2. *Collecting system and ureter*
   • Dilatation (hydronephrosis and hydroureter)
   • Non-calcified stone or tumor (black filling defect)
   • Laceration (leaking of contrast; Fig.4-3).
3. *Bladder contour*

Remember to always compare the contrast injected films with the scout film, by looking at them back and forth (Fig.4-4). The contrast injected films are used to determine if a calcification seen on the scout film is inside or outside of a ureter (Fig.4-5).

III. Specific problems

A. Hydronephrosis and hydroureter

Imagine that one of the kids obstructs his straw with a pebble, or by pinching it. He needs a deeper breath to overcome the obstruction. When blowing, his face becomes red and the air flow in his straw is slow. Both the straw before the obstruction and the kid's cheeks dilate because of back pressure (Fig.4-1B). This situation is analogous to an obstructing ureteric stone (pebble) or a tumor encasing the ureter (pinching).

On the IVP, look for the following signs of obstruction (Fig.4-6A, 4-6B, 4-6C, 4-6D).

1. *Delayed nephrogram and delayed contrast excretion:* The affected kidney and collecting system take longer to brighten (deeper breath, slow air flow).
2. *Hyperdense nephrogram:* The affected kidney becomes too white (red face).
3. *Hydronephrosis* (Fig.4-7) and *hydroureter*. Dilation of the collecting system (blown up cheeks) and dilatation of the ureter (dilated straw) before the obstruction.

Initial films may not show the site of obstruction since it takes longer to outline a blocked system with contrast. Therefore, to locate the site of obstruction, one *must* ask for delayed films. To do this, double the time of the last film. For example, if the last film was taken at 30 minutes after injection, ask for a 1 hour film.

Remember that hydronephrosis and hydroureter may be caused by something other than an obstruction (e.g. *Reflux nephropathy*). When there is no delayed nephrogram and no delayed contrast excretion, there is no obstruction.

B. No nephrogram

Imagine that the blushing face of one kid is not visible. It either means that he is not blowing or that he is not there. Similarly, when there is no nephrogram on one side, either the kidney is non-functioning (Fig. 4-1C) or it is absent (Fig. 4-1D)

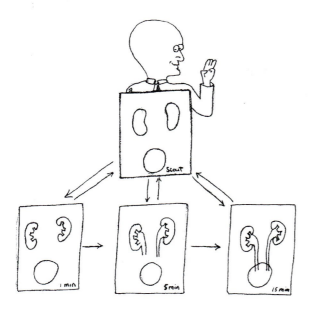

Fig.4-4: Search pattern. Always compare the contrast injected films with the scout film by looking at them back and forth.

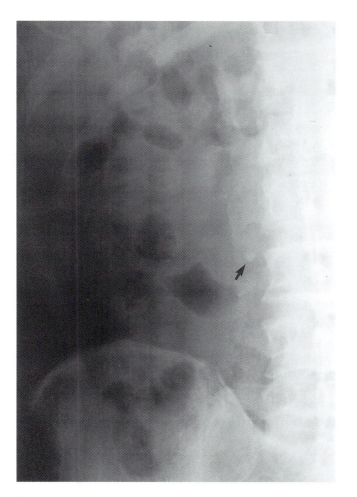

A

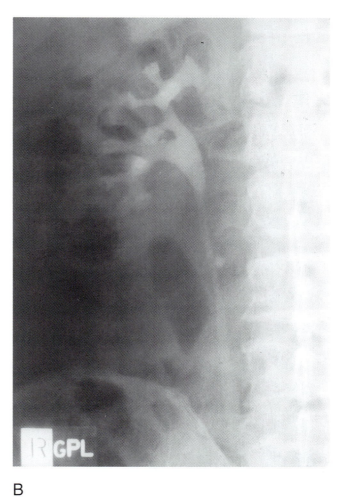

B

Fig.4-5: Calcification outside the ureter. A. Magnified view of a scout film showing a calcification (black arrow), which appears to be a right ureteric stone. B. Magnified view of a contrast injected film showing that calcification is outside of the right ureter and therefore is not a ureteric stone.

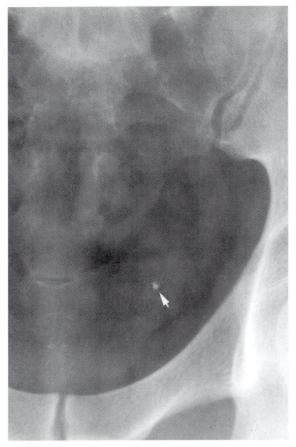

A

B

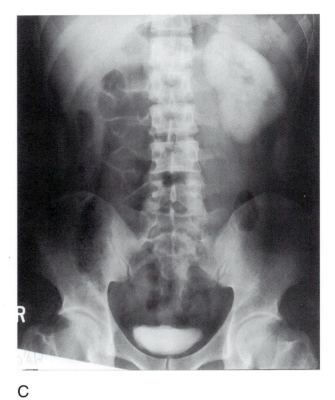

C

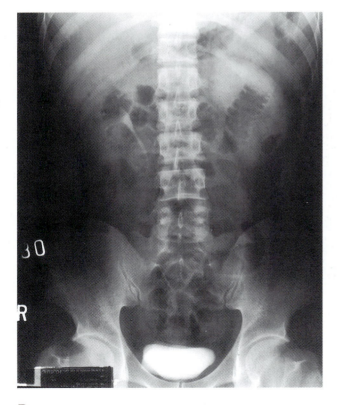

D

Fig.4-6: Left obstructing ureteric stone.   A. Magnified view of a scout film showing a tiny stone (arrow head), which could be located in the distal left ureter. B. 30 minute film showing normal contrast excretion of the right kidney and hyperdense left nephrogram. C. 2 hour and a half film shows complete contrast clearance of the right kidney. However the left nephrogram is still hyperdense. D. 7 hour and a half film showing delayed excretion of contrast into the left ureter.

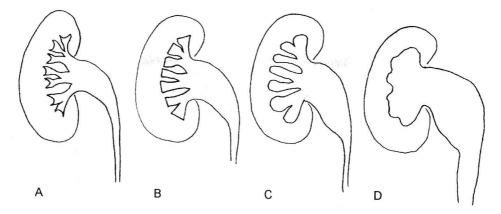

Fig.4-7: Hydronephrosis. A. Normal pelvicalyceal system. B. mild hydronephrosis. C. moderate hydronephrosis D. Severe hydronephrosis. and *hydroureter:* Dilatation of the collecting system (blown up cheeks) and dilatation of the ureter (dilated straw) before the obstruction.

Chapter 5.   Cervical Spine

I. Radiographic anatomy

Imagine a Greek statue representing the Titan "Atlas" who is supporting the earth's weight as a punishment by Zeus (Fig.5-1). The Titan is sitting on a stool on top of a Greek column. The work is made of 7 marble blocks. The top one is sculpted into Atlas. The block under Atlas includes a stool, which serves as a supporting axis for the statue. Atlas's massive feet rest on the edges of this second block. All other blocks are cemented one on top of each other to make a column.

The cervical spine is structured in much the same way as the above Greek statue. 7 cervical vertebrae numbered 1 to 7, from top to bottom, are stacked on top of each other to make a column (Fig.5-2). The top vertebra, which supports the head's weight, is called *Atlas* (C1) after the famous Titan. It lies on *Axis* (C2), which has a stool-like protrusion called the *odontoid process*. In reality, Atlas surrounds the odontoid process without technically sitting on it. Much like the Titan's massive feet, Atlas' *lateral masses* rest on the edges of Axis (Fig.5-3). In addition, this column is held in

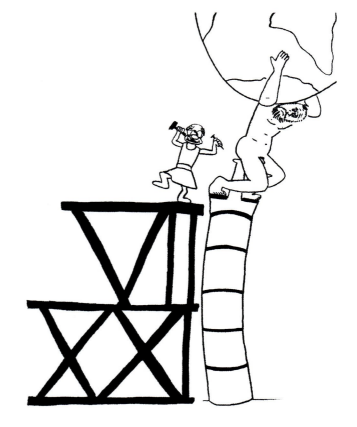

Fig.5-1:   Atlas on a Greek column.   Restoration of the statue of Atlas on a Greek column is analogous to the cervical spine. The roman numbers 7 and 21 in the scaffold help remember that the prevertebral soft tissue thickness should measure no greater than 7mm at the C3 level and no greater than 21 mm at the C7 level.

place by several ligaments, and each vertebra is separated by cement-like spacers (the *intervertebral disks*). Notice the cervical column is slightly curved posteriorly (*lordosis*).

A typical cervical vertebra has a body, two transverse and one spinous process, two transverse and one vertebral foramen. Surrounding the vertebral foramen are two pedicles, two lateral masses and two laminae (Fig.5-4). The lateral

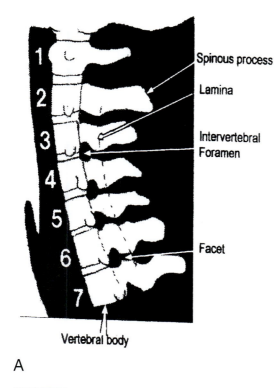

Spinous process

Lamina

Intervertebral Foramen

Facet

Vertebral body

A

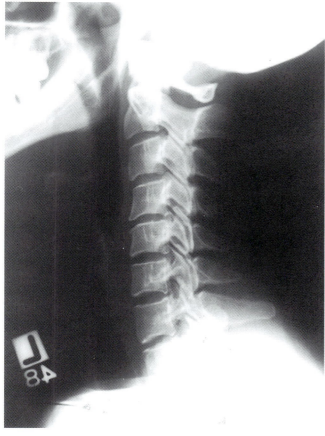

B

Fig.5-2:   Lateral view of the normal cervical spine.   A. Diagram. B. Radiograph.

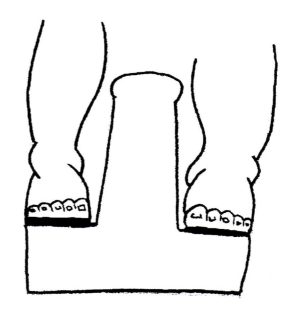

A

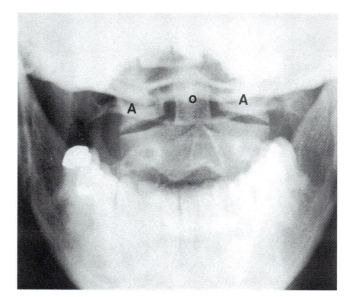

B

Fig.5-3:   Open mouth view.   A. Atlas sits on Axis' stool-like protrusion called the odontoid process. Atlas' massive feet rest on the edges of Axis. B. Similarly, the lateral masses of Atlas (A) rest on the Axis' edges. Odontoid process (O).

masses support the facet articular surfaces, which enable the vertebrae to articulate with each other. The vertebral arteries run through the transverse foramina and the spinal cord runs through the vertebral foramen.

The ancient statue is in need of restoration. Therefore, a scaffold has been placed in front of it. Analogous with the scaffold, there is soft tissue in front of the vertebral column (*prevertebral soft tissue*).

II. Approach

You are "Jefferson" a famous architect. Help the Greek sculptor (Cervicos Spinos) to restore the ancient column of Atlas by applying the following principles:

1. Look at the column from different angles (e.g. frontal and lateral views). Ensure that the entire column, including the foundation, is visible.
2. Look at the alignment between the blocks.
3. Look for cracks in each individual block. Inspect the cement between each blocks
4. Ensure that the scaffold is adequate.
5. Look especially at the stool and Atlas' massive feet.

In much the same way, C-spine films include a *lateral,* a *frontal* and *Open-Mouth view* to assess the following:

A. Lateral view

This film is the most important one. It must be examined methodically so that no area is forgotten. On this film, look for:

1. Ensure that 7 vertebral bodies are seen:

If the seventh cervical vertebra is not completely visible, a *swimmer's* view may be obtained. This view is a lateral view with one of the patient's arms raised, to display C7 more clearly.

2. Alignment:

Make sure that all cervical vertebrae align properly, by drawing 4 imaginary lines (Fig.5-5). Ensure that these lines are continuous and that no *step-deformity* is present, which could represent a dislocation of the facet joints or a fracture. The most reliable and important of these lines is the posterior vertebral line, because it is least often disrupted by bony spurs seen with aging (*osteophytes*), and because it is directly adjacent to the spinal cord.

3. Bones:

Look for any fractures. Measure the distance between the odontoid process and the anterior portion of the atlas (C1). If this measurement is >3mm (Fig.5-6), a fracture or a dislocation at this site is suspected, and CT confirmation is needed.

4. Cartilage:

Look for markedly decreased intervertebral disc space. This may be secondary to *degenerative disc disease* (wear and tear).

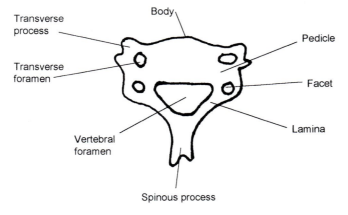

Fig.5-4: **Normal cervical vertebra.**

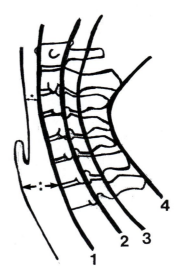

Fig.5-5: **Normal alignment of cervical vertebrae and normal prevertebral soft tissues.**   Four imaginary lines are used to assess cervical spine alignment as follows: the anterior vertebral line (number one), the posterior vertebral line (number two), the spino-laminar line (number three) and the spinous process line (number four). Also, the normal soft tissue thickness at the C2-C3 level is less then seven mm (one star) and at the C6-C7 level is less than 21 mm (two stars).

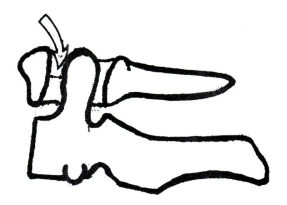

A

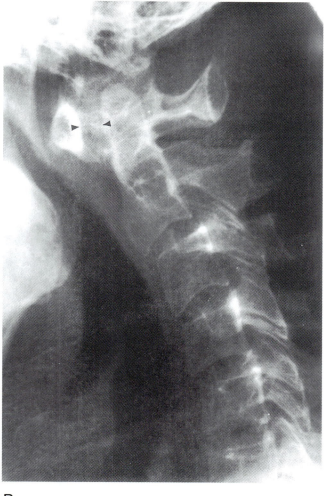

B

5. Soft tissues:

Look for prevertebral soft tissue enlargement, which is suggestive of soft tissue swelling or hematoma. The prevertebral soft tissue should measure no greater than 7mm at the C3 level and no greater than 21 mm at the C7 level (Fig.5-5, 5-1). Even when measurements are normal, a focal bulge is always suggestive of soft tissue swelling or hematoma. Ensure that the airway is not compromised.

B. Frontal view

Often the highest vertebrae are difficult to see in this view. Ensure that no major discontinuity is present, that all spinous processes are aligned, that there are no fractures, that the disc spaces are preserved and that there is no large soft tissue mass (Fig.5-7).

C. Odontoid view (Open-mouth view)

Ensure that the edges of the lateral masses of the Atlas are perfectly aligned with the edges of the Axis. Slippage of the lateral masses sideways is suggestive of a fracture.

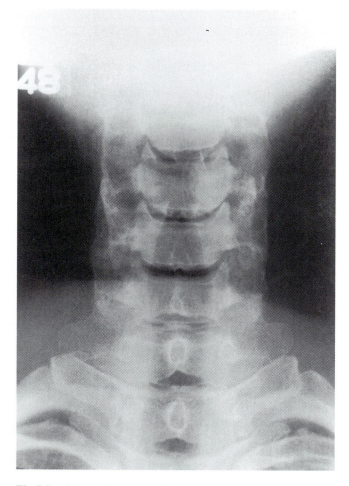

Fig.5-6: Normal anterior atlanto-odontoid space. A. The normal space between the anterior part of C1 and the odontoid process is less than 3 mm (empty arrow). B. Magnified lateral radiograph of the cervical spine showing abnormal increased space (5 mm) between the anterior part of C1 and the odontoid process (arrow heads).

Fig.5-7:   Normal frontal radiograph of the cervical spine.

Also, look for any black line across the odontoid process, which would suggest a fracture (Fig.5-3, 5-13).

III. Specific problems

A. Dislocations

1. Atlantooccipital dislocation (unstable)

Atlantooccipital dislocation is analogous to the Titan Atlas dropping the earth. It is a dislocation at the junction between the Atlas vertebra and the skull. This unstable entity is caused by a complex injury and often results in death. The anterior dislocation is much more frequent and much easier to see on X-ray. It usually gives rise to an increase in prevertebral soft tissue width (hematoma; Fig.5-8).

2. Facet joint dislocations (unstable)

Facet dislocation is analogous to misaligned blocks in our Greek column. It is best seen on the lateral view as a step deformity within the vertebral alignment. A step deformity of >3mm is always abnormal and means that the spine is unstable. Facet dislocation occurs secondarily to hyperflexion of the cervical spine. This hyperflexion results in disruption of the anterior longitudinal ligament (which lies anterior to the vertebral body), intervertebral disc, and posterior ligaments.

There are 3 types of bilateral facet dislocations, all of which are unstable. They are, in order of increasing severity, the *subluxed facets,* the *perched facets,* and *locked facets* (Fig.5-9).

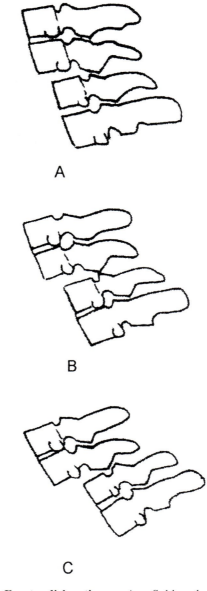

A

B

C

Fig.5-9: Facet dislocations: A. Subluxed facets. B. Perched facets. C. Locked facets. D. Lateral radiograph showing anterior displacement (black arrow) of C4 over C5. The facets at this level are subluxed (white arrow). E. Lateral radiograph showing anterior displacement (black arrow) of C4 over C5. One facet pair is perched (white arrow) while the other is locked (white arrow head) .

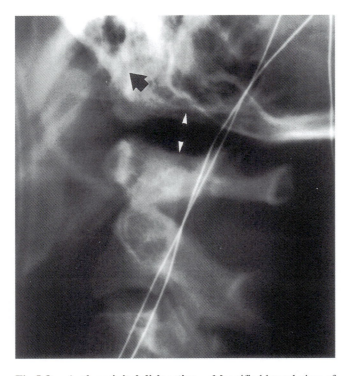

Fig.5-8: Antlooccipital dislocation. Magnified lateral view of the upper cervical spine showing increased distance between Atlas and the skull (white arrow heads). There is also anterior displacement of the skull in relation to the spine (black arrow).

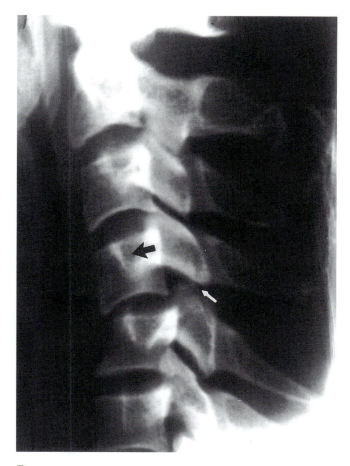

D

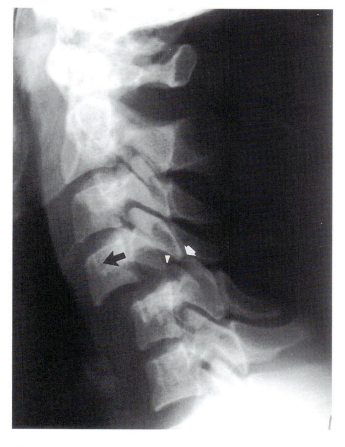

E

Fig.5-9 *(continued)*

B. Fractures

1. Unstable

a. Flexion Teardrop

This fracture is secondary to a flexion injury. It is extremely unstable and severe, and therefore should not be confused with the more benign extension teardrop fracture. It results in disruption of all ligaments as well as the intervertebral disc at the level of injury. A small fragment of the anteroinferior portion is broken off of a vertebral body with posterior displacement of the vertebral body itself. This type of fracture often results in anterior spinal cord compression (Fig.5-10A).

b. Hangman's

This fracture is secondary to a extension injury, which commonly occurs in motor vehicle accidents (MVA) or in hangings (hence the name). It is a bilateral C2 pedicle fracture, with anterior displacement of the anterior part of C2 (Fig.5-10B, 5-11).

c. Hyperextension Fracture-Dislocation

This fracture is secondary to an extension injury and is unstable. It results in a slight anterior vertebral subluxation, with a complex fracture near the articular surfaces (fig.5-10C).

d. Burst

This unstable fracture results from an axial injury. It is a compression of the vertebral body and results in loss of both anterior and posterior vertebral body height. This is unlike the wedge fracture, in which there is only loss of anterior vertebral body height. Bony fragments may push on the spinal cord and cause symptoms. This type of fracture is most commonly located in the mid-cervical spine (Fig.5-10D).

e. Jefferson's

A Jefferson's fracture consists of at least two fractures of C1. A ring structure cannot be broken in only one spot. Try breaking a lifesaver in only one spot, it's impossible! This unstable fracture is secondary to an axial injury. Examples of

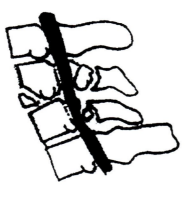

A

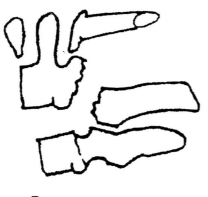

B

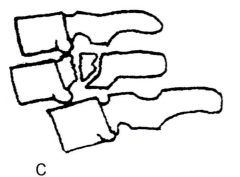

C

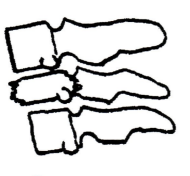

D

Fig.5-10: **Drawing of unstable fractures.** A. Flexion teardrop. B. Hangman's. C. Hyperextension fracture dislocation. D. Burst

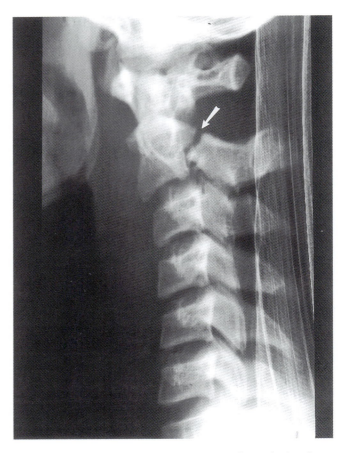

Fig.5-11: **Hangman's fracture.** Lateral radiograph showing a fracture through the pedicles of C2 (white arrow).

axial injuries include having a heavy object fall on one's head or diving into an empty pool.

Jefferson's fracture is analogous to Atlas' massive feet slipping off the edges of the second block. Look at the open mouth view to see if the Atlas' lateral masses have slipped sideways and therefore are no longer flush with the Axis edges (Fig.5-12).

f. Odontoid

An odontoid fracture is analogous to a crack in the Titan's stool. Look at the open-mouth view for a black line in the odontoid process, which would represent a fracture. This unstable fracture is secondary to a multidirectional injury and is a fracture of the odontoid process of C2. There are three types of odontoid fractures, the most unstable of which is type 2 (Fig.5-13).

2. Stable

a. Clay-Shoveler's

This stable fracture is secondary to a flexion injury. It involves an avulsion of a piece of the spinous process and most

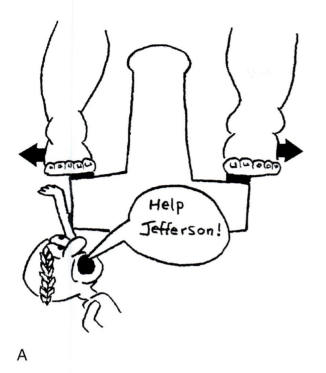

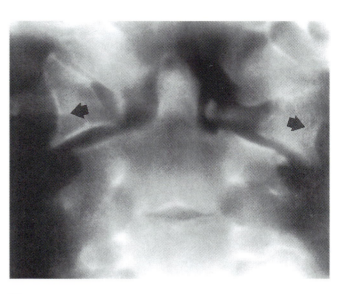

A

B

Fig.5-12: Jefferson's fracture. Atlas' massive feet representing the Atlas' (C1) lateral masses slip laterally and are no longer at the edges of Axis (C2).

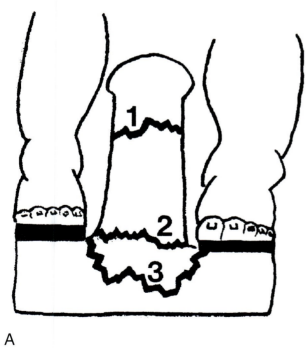

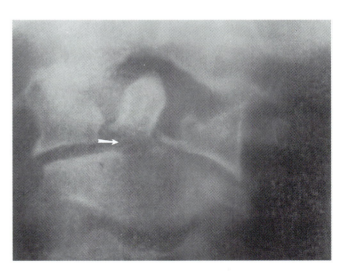

A

B

Fig.5-13: Odontoid fractures. A. Type 1,2,and 3 odontoid fractures. B. Open mouth radiograph showing a type 2 odontoid fracture (white arrow).

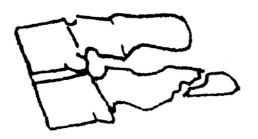

A

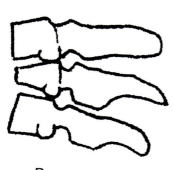

B

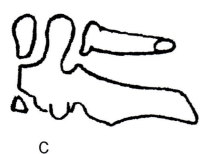

C

Fig.5-14: Drawing of stable fractures. A. Clay shoveler's. B. Wedge. C. Extension teardrop.

frequently occurs in the lower C-spine. It is best seen on the lateral view (Fig.5-14A, 5-15).

b. Wedge

This stable fracture is the result of a flexion injury. It involves compression of the anterior part of the verte-

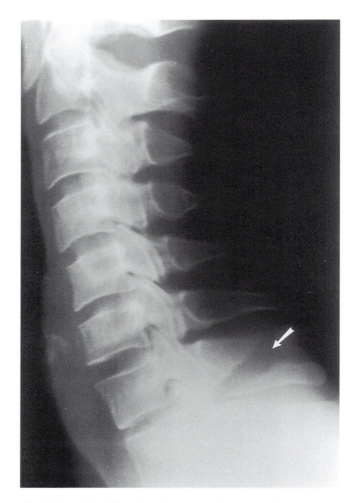

Fig.5-15: Clay Shoveler's fracture. Lateral radiograph showing a fracture (white arrow) of C7's spinous process.

bral body and therefore is best seen on the lateral view (Fig.5-14B).

c. Extension Teardrop

This stable fracture is the result of an extension injury. It is an avulsion of a piece of the anteroinferior portion of a vertebra and often occurs at C2 (Fig.5-14C).

Chapter 6.   Axial Skeleton

I. Radiographic anatomy

A. Skull

Several different views are useful to look at specific parts of the skull optimally. *Caldwell, Waters* and the *lateral* views are most frequently used.

1. Caldwell view

A Caldwell view is a frontal radiograph of the head taken with the patient's face against the film (PA). This view best displays the frontal sinuses, the orbital rim and the medial orbital wall. The maxillary, the ethmoid and the sphenoid sinuses are often more difficult to assess because of overlap with other structures (Fig.6-1A) The skull sutures, the zygo-matic bones, the nasal bones, the nasal septum and the mandible are also seen.

2. Waters view

A Waters view is a PA radiograph of the skull with the patient's head tilted back (much like someone drinking water!). This view displays best the orbital rim, the floor of the orbit, the maxillary sinuses, the zygomatic bones, the nasal septum and nasal bones (fig.6-1B).

3. Lateral view

A lateral view of the skull is a radiograph of the patient in profile. This view best displays the ethmoid and sphenoid sinuses (Fig.6-1C).

51

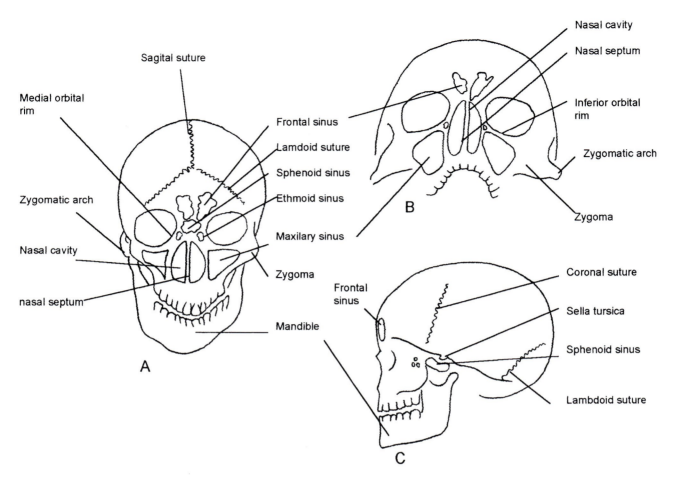

Fig.6-1:   Skull anatomy.   A. Caldwell view. B. Waters view. C. Lateral view.

B. Thoracolumbar spine

The thoracic spine is composed of 12 vertebrae, which are numbered T1 to T12 from top to bottom. The vertebrae are separated by intervertebral disks much like the cervical spine. The thoracic spine is concave anteriorly (*kyphosis*). The lumbar spine is composed of 5 vertebrae called L1 to L5, again from top to bottom (Fig.6-2A). It is concave posteriorly (*lordosis*), like the cervical spine.

A typical vertebra is composed of a body, two transverse processes, pedicles, pars interarticularis, laminae and one spinous process. In the center is the vertebral foramen, which contains the spinal cord (Fig.6-3).

On the frontal view of the spine, each vertebra looks like an owl. Each eye represents a pedicle and the beak of the owl represents the spinous process (Fig.6-2B).

When a radiograph of the spine is taken obliquely, each vertebra takes on the appearance of a Scottie dog! Each part of the dog correspond to a component of the the vertebra (Fig.6-2C). The front legs and hind legs represent the inferior intervertebral articular processes, the ears and the tail are the superior intervertebral articular processes. Therefore, the Scottie dogs are standing on each others ears and tails to form the intervertebral articulation. The body of the Scottie dog corresponds to one of the laminae, the eye is one of the pedicles, the nose is one of the transverse processes, and the neck is the *pars interarticularis*. If the behind of the Scottie dog is located to the right, you are looking at the right lamina, pars interarticularis and pedicle, and vice versa.

C. Pelvis

The pelvis is just like a pretzel. It is composed of three rings, which are one central pelvic inlet, and two obturator canals (Fig.6-4). The pelvic inlet is composed of the sacral bone, the iliac bones and the pubic bones. The pubic bones, which are fused to the iliac bones, articulate with each other at the pubic symphysis. The sacrum articulates with the two iliac bones at the sacroiliac (SI) joints. The obtrator canals are composed of the pubic rami superiorly and ischial rami inferiorly.

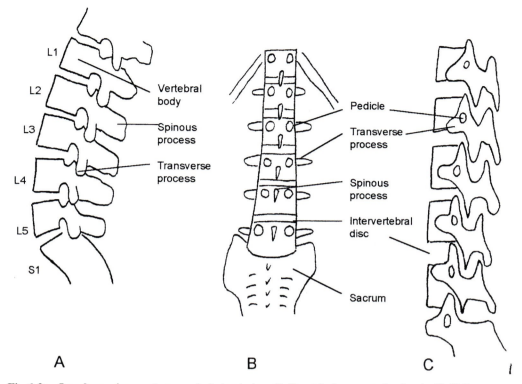

Fig.6-2: Lumbar spine anatomy. A. Lateral view. B. Frontal view: stack of owls. C. Oblique view: stack of scottie dogs.

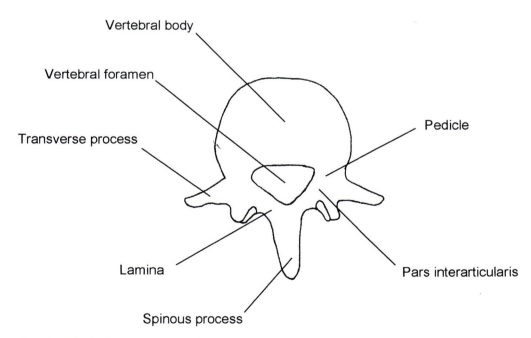

Fig.6-3: Typical lumbar vertebra.

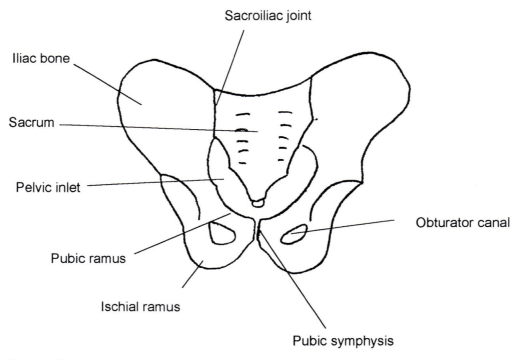

Fig.6-4: Pelvic anatomy.

II. Approach

A. Skull

There are four types of dark line on a skull radiograph (Fig.6-5):

1. Large sinuous: Grooves in which arteries run.
2. Small sinuous: Suture lines.
3. Zigzag : Fracture.
4. Straight: Fracture.

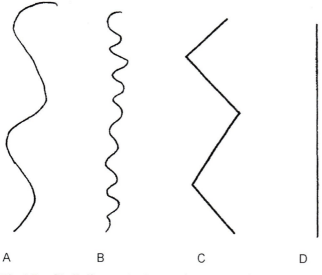

Fig.6-5: Skull lines.   A. Large sinuous. B. Small sinuous. C. Zigzag. D. Straight.

There are 3 views of the skull frequently used:

1. Caldwell view

Look at the orbital rim and the medial orbital wall for any fracture lines. Also ensure that the sinuses are of air density (black) and do not contain any fluid density material (white). Fluid in the sinuses could represent blood from a nearby fracture or fluid from sinusitis.

2. Waters view

Look at the orbital rim, orbital floor, nasal bones and septum for fractures. Ensure that the sinuses (especially the maxillary sinuses) do not contain fluid density material (white).

3. Lateral view

Look at the skull for any fracture line and at the ethmoid and sphenoid sinuses for any abnormal fluid.

B. Thoracolumbar spine

1. Frontal view

On the frontal view, the thoracolumbar spine looks like owls' heads piled on one another.

• Look at the pile of owl's heads for any step-deformity (misalignment of the spine).
• Ensure that the distance between each head is equal (intervertebral disk space)

- Look at each owl's face for:
  - missing eye (destruction of a pedicle)
  - crack in the eye (see Chance fracture)
  - increased space between the eyes (see Burst fracture)
  - decreased head's height (see Burst fracture)
  - open owl's beak or increase distance between 2 beaks.(see Chance and spinous process fractures)

2. Lateral view

- Look at the alignment of the vertebrae.
- Ensure that the intervertebral disk spaces are even throughout.
- Compare the anterior and posterior cortex of each vertebral body for any differences in height with adjacent ones (specific fractures discussed later).
- Look for any black fracture lines in the spinous processes.

3. Oblique view

The oblique view of the thoracolumbar spine looks like a pile of Scottie dogs. Ensure none of them has a collar, which implies pars interarticularis defect (see Spondylolysis section).

C. Pelvis

On the frontal view, the pelvis looks like a pretzel. Remember that a pretzel ring never breaks at only one place.

Therefore, after finding a fracture in one of the pelvic rings, one *must* look for a second fracture line.

- Compare one side of the pretzel with the other.
- Look for any black fracture lines in all three pretzel rings.
- Look for any widening of the SI joints and pubic symphysis.
- Look for black fracture lines in the iliac wings and sacrum.

III. Specific problems

A. Skull

1. Blow out orbital fracture

A blow out orbital fracture occurs when there is sudden increase in intraorbital pressure (e.g. receiving a squash ball in the eye). The eye has nowhere to go and is pushed against the bony structures of the orbital cavity. This usually results in fracture or "blow out" of the orbital floor (weakest portion of the orbit), although the medial wall may also blow out.

Look at the Caldwell and Waters views for bony fragments in the superior aspect of the maxillary sinuses (Fig.6-6). Also look for air in the orbit or fluid (blood) in the maxillary sinuses and ethmoid sinuses.

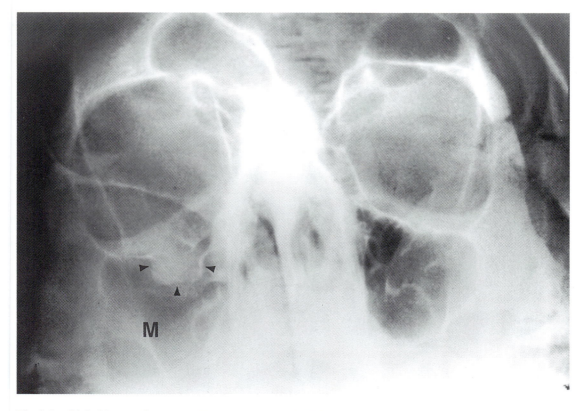

Fig.6-6: Right blow out fracture.   Waters view of the skull showing soft tissue (arrow heads) from the right orbit in the right maxillary sinus (M). It has herniated through a fracture in the orbital floor.

2. Zygomatic arch fracture

a. Simple

Simple zygomatic arch fractures can be seen on the Caldwell or the Waters view. They are usually the result of a blow to the zygomatic arch and are less frequent than tripod fractures (described below).

b. Tripod

A tripod fracture is a combination 3 fractures. The fractures are typically located at the zygomatic arch, the frontozygomatic and the maxillozygomatic sutures (Fig.6-7). This triple fracture results in having a free floating zygomatic bone.

3. Nasal fracture

Nasal fractures occur most frequently in the lower portion of the nasal bone and are often associated with nasal septum fractures. The fracture fragment is often displaced towards the nasal cavity. This injury is frequently the result of a mild to moderate frontal impact (punch on the nose).

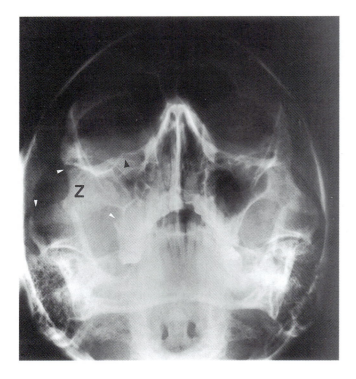

Fig.6-7: Right tripod fracture. Waters view showing a zygomatic arch fracture, a frontozygomatic fracture and a maxillozygomatic fracture (white arrow heads). The right zygoma (Z) is therefore free floating. In addition, there is a right inferior orbital rim fracture (black arrow head). The right maxillary sinus contains blood and therefore appears whiter than the one on the left.

4. Le Fort fractures

Major facial fractures are classified using the Le Fort system, which is composed of three types (Fig.6-8). The mechanism of injury is severe frontal impact (face hits the dash board in a car accident).

Le Fort type 1:   This fracture results in separation of the palate from the rest of the face and gives rise to a floating palate. The fracture line goes through the maxillary bones and the nasal septum.

Le Fort type 2:   This fracture results in separation of the maxillary bone from the rest of the face and therefore gives rise to a floating maxilla. The fracture line goes through the maxillary sinuses, inferior and medial orbital rims, and the nose.

Le Fort type 3:   This fracture results in the separation of the entire face from the rest of the skull, which gives rise to a floating face. The fracture line goes through the zygomatic arches, the lateral and medial orbital rims and the nose.

5. Mandibular fracture

Mandibular fractures often occur at the body, the angle or the neck (Fig.6-9).

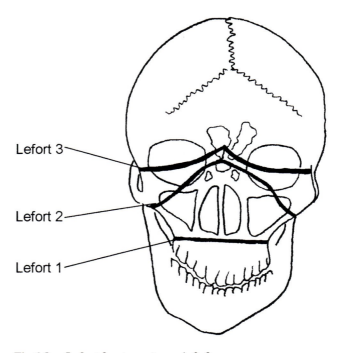

Fig.6-8:   Lefort fractures types 1, 2, 3.

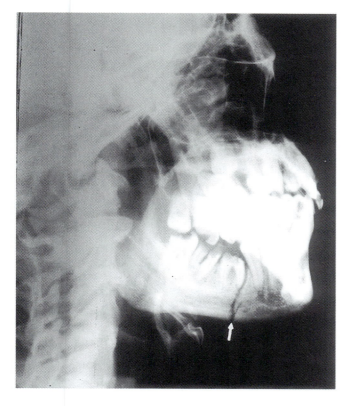

Fig.6-9: **Mandibular fracture (white arrow).**

B. Thoracolumbar spine

1. Unstable injury

a. Chance fracture

A chance fracture results in horizontal severing of a vertebra (Fig.6-10A). Chance fractures are best seen on a lateral view of the spine (Fig.6-10B). Sometimes when the fracture line extends through the spinous process, one can see the two distinct pieces on the frontal view. It looks like there are two spinous processes at one level (like if the beak of the owl at the affected level is open; Fig.6-10C, 6-10D). This unstable injury is often the result of a *Motor Vehicle Accident (MVA)* where a lap belt immobilizes the pelvis, while the rest of the upper body is thrust forward.

b. Burst fracture

A burst fracture results in collapse of an entire vertebral body. On a lateral view, the height of the anterior and posterior wall of the vertebral body are smaller in comparison to adjacent normal vertebrae (Fig.6-11A, 6-11B). Fragments extending into the spinal canal are common and may cause neurological damage. On the frontal view, the interpedicular distance is increased. The mechanism of injury is fall from a height.

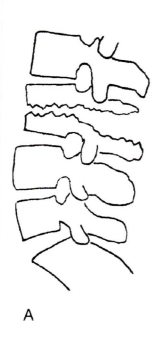

A

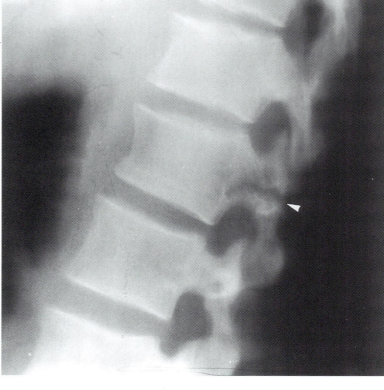

B

Fig.6-10: **Chance fracture.** A. Lateral view of a Chance fracture showing horizontal severing of a vertebra. B. Lateral lumbar spine radiograph of a Chance fracture. C. Frontal view of a Chance fracture showing a crack in the pedicles (eyes of the owl), and in the spinous process (open beak of the owl). D. Frontal lumbar spine radiograph of a Chance fracture.

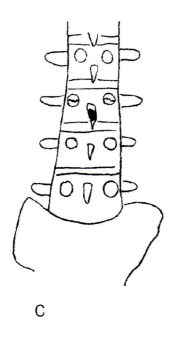

C

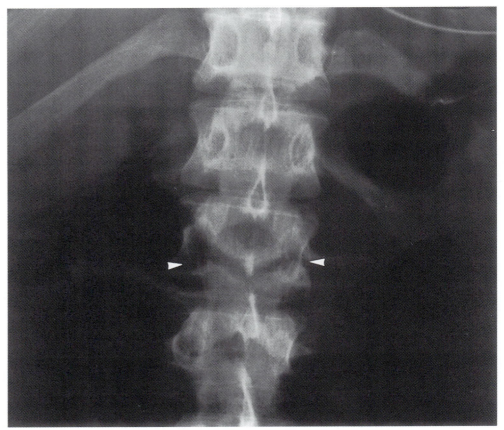

Fig.6-10: (*continued*) D

2. Stable injury

a. Wedge fracture

A wedge fracture results in the collapse of the anterior vertebral body. On the lateral view, there is decreased height of the anterior wall of the vertebral body in comparison to adjacent normal vertebrae. The posterior wall of the vertebral body is intact. The spinal canal is not involved and there is no neurological damage. A wedge fracture is a hyperflexion injury.

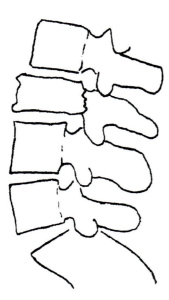

A

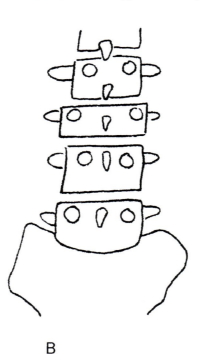

B

Fig.6-11: Burst fracture. A. Lateral view of a burst fracture showing both posterior and anterior vertebral wall compression. B. Frontal view of a burst fracture showing a widened interpedicular space (space between an owl's eyes).

b. Spinous process fracture

In this injury, there is a black fracture line in the spinous process. The spinal canal and the stability of the spine are unaffected.

c. Spondylolysis

Spondylolysis is usually a defect in the pars interarticularis. It is best seen on oblique view where it appears as a collar on a Scottie dog (Fig.6-12A). Spondylolysis is most often seen at the L4 or L5 level.

d. Spondylolisthesis

Spondylolisthesis occurs when there are bilateral pars interarticularis defects (bilateral spondylolysis).The vertebral body of the affected level is only held against the rest of the vertebra by ligaments and intervertebral disc. With time, this superior vertebral body slips forward on the inferior one. This anterior subluxation is classified into four grades, which indicates the percentage of displacement (Fig.6-12B, 6-12C, 6-12D, 6-12E).

C. Pelvis

1. Unstable injury

Unstable pelvic fractures occur less often than the stable ones but are associated with significant pelvic organ trauma, hemorrhage and shock.

a. Malgaigne fracture

A Malgaigne fracture often involves fractures through the ischiopubic rami (or the pubic symphysis) and the SI joint of the same side. Fracture fragments can be displaced vertically (Fig.6-13A, 6-14).

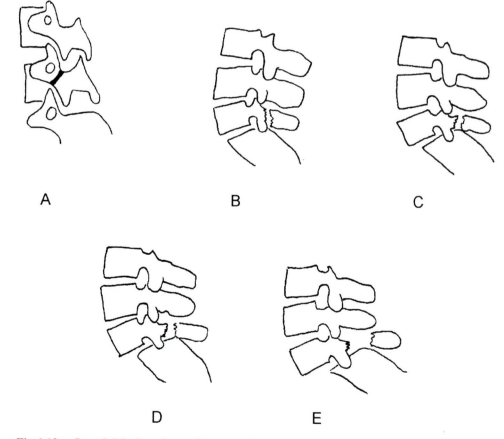

A   B   C

D   E

Fig.6-12: Spondylolysis and spondylolysthesis. A. Spondylolysis. Oblique view of the lumbar spine showing a pars interarticularis defect (collar on Scottie dog). B. Grade 1 spondylolysthesis C. Grade 2 spondylolysthesis. D. Grade 3 spondylolysthesis. E. Grade 4 spondylolysthesis.

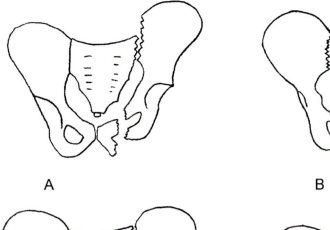
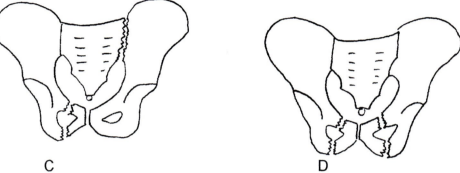

Fig.6-13: Unstable pelvic fractures.   A. Malgaigne fracture. B. Open book fracture. C. Bucket handle fracture. D. Straddle fracture.

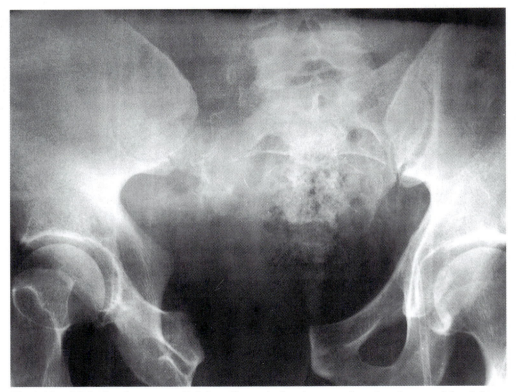

Fig.6-14: Malgaine fracture.   Pelvic radiograph showing complete detachment of the right hemipelvis.

b. Open book fracture

An open book fracture often involves fractures through the ischiopubic rami (or pubic symphysis) and SI joints on both sides. The pelvis is cracked open like a book (Fig.6-13B).

c. Bucket handle fracture

A bucket handle fracture often involves fractures through the ischiopubic rami on one side and SI joint fracture is on the opposite side (Fig.6-13C).

d. Straddle fracture

A straddle fracture goes through both ischial rami and pubic rami (Fig.6-13D, 6-15). The small piece of bone containing the pubic symphysis is free to move.

2. Stable injury

a. Rami fractures

Rami fractures are located at both the ischial ramus and pubic ramus, and are stable.

b. Avulsion fracture

An avulsion fracture occurs when a small chip of bone is pulled off at the origin or insertion site of a tendon.

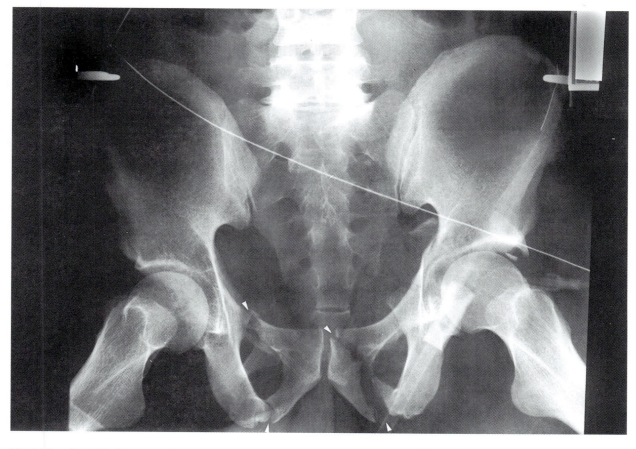

Fig.6-15: Straddle fracture. Pelvic radiograph showing fractures through both ischial and pubic rami (arrow heads).

Chapter 7.   Limbs

I. Radiographic anatomy
    A. Terminology
    B. Upper limb
        1. Shoulder
        2. Arm
        3. Elbow
        4. Forearm
        5. Wrist
        6. Hand
    C. Lower limb
        1. Hip
        2. Thigh
        3. Knee
        4. Leg
        5. Ankle
        6. Foot
II. Approach
III. Specific problems
    A. Upper limb
        1. Shoulder
            a. Proximal humeral fracture
            b. Glenohumeral joint dislocation
            c. Acromioclavicular joint separation
            d. Clavicular fracture
        2. Humeral shaft fracture
        3. Elbow
            a. Distal humeral fracture
            b. Proximal ulna fracture
            c. Elbow dislocation
            d. Radial head fracture
        4. Forearm
            a. Monteggia fracture-dislocation
            b. Galeazzi fracture-dislocation
        5. Wrist
            a. Colles' fracture
            b. Smith's fracture
            c. Scaphoid fracture
            d. Wrist dislocations
        6. Hand
            a. First metacarpal base fractures
            b. Skier's thumb
            c. Boxer's fracture
            d. Baseball finger
    B. Lower limb
        1. Hip
            a. Hip fractures
            b. Hip dislocations
        2. Femoral shaft fracture

3. Knee
   a. Tibial plateau fracture
   b. Patellar fracture
4. Tibial and fibular fractures
5. Ankle fracture
6. Foot
   a. Calcaneal fracture
   b. March fracture
   c. Jones' fracture

I. Radiographic anatomy

A. Terminology

Anatomical position: Visualize the human body with the palms of the hands and the back of the feet forward.

Midline: Central vertical axis of the body.

Medial: Close to the midline.

Lateral: Away from the midline.

Proximal: Closer to the head.

Distal: Further from the head.

Palmar (volar): Palm side of the hand.

Plantar: Under side of the foot.

Dorsal: Back side of the hand and foot.

Abduction: Movement of a joint away from midline.

Adduction: Movement of a joint close to midline.

Pronation: Forearm moving from anatomical position to palm facing posterior.

Supination: Forearm moving from palm facing posteriorly back into anatomical position (palm facing forward).

Epiphysis: End part of a long bone.

Diaphysis: Middle part of a long bone (shaft).

Metaphysis: Funnel-shaped part of a long bone between the epiphysis and the diaphysis.

Cortex: Outer portion of the bone.

Intraarticular: Inside the joint.

Extraarticular: Outside the joint.

B. Upper limb

1. Shoulder

The shoulder (Fig.7-1A) is composed of 3 joints. The scapula is a triangular flat bone. At its lateral aspect, it has a

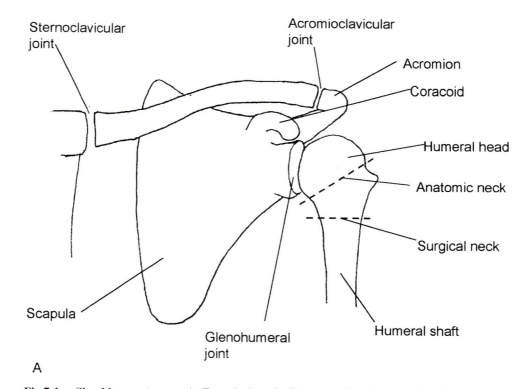

Fig.7-1: Shoulder anatomy. A. Frontal view. B. Trans-scapular view showing the Mercedez Benz sign.

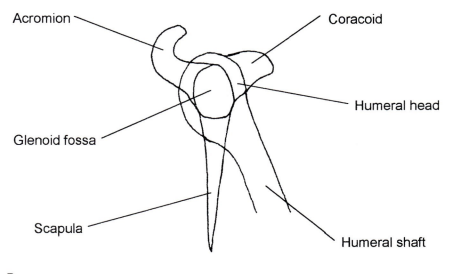

B

Fig.7-1: Shoulder anatomy. A. Frontal view. B. Trans-scapular view showing the Mercedez Benz sign.

cup-like structure called the glenoid fossa, which articulates with the humeral head (*glenohumeral joint*). Also, located laterally are two hook-like structures called the acromion (superior) and the coracoid process (inferior). The "S" shaped clavicle articulates with both the acromion (*acromioclavicular joint*) and the sternum (*sternoclavicular joint*). The anatomical and surgical necks of the humerus are located distal to the humeral head.

The scapula has a bony ridge (spine) running on its posterior aspect. On the lateral view of the scapula (*transscapular view;* Fig.7-1B), this arrangement normally gives the appearance of the *Mercedes Benz sign.* The round humeral head is normally located in the center of this sign.

2. Arm (humeral shaft)

The humeral shaft is a tube-like structure. Remember that the radial nerve runs behind it.

3. Elbow

The distal humerus has two distal articular surfaces or condyles, which are called *capitellum* and *trochlea,* lying laterally and medially respectively (Fig.7-2). Capitellum means head in latin. For this reason, it is not surprising that it articulates with the head of the radius. In contrast, the trochlea rests in the *trochlear notch* of the ulna. Just anterior to this

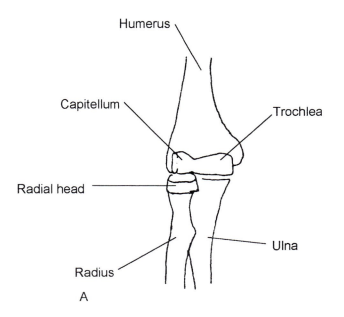

A

Fig.7-2: Elbow anatomy. A. Frontal view. B. Lateral view.

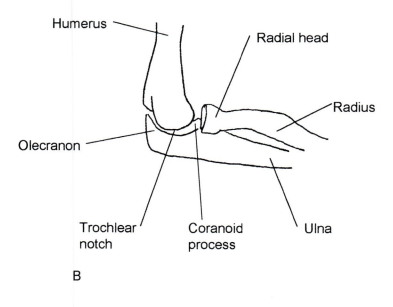

Humerus
Radial head
Radius
Olecranon
Trochlear notch
Coranoid process
Ulna

B

Fig.7-2: (*continued*)

notch is a small bony protrusion called the *coronoid process* of the ulna and just posterior to this notch is the pointy bony part of the elbow tip called the *olecranon process* of the ulna.

4. Forearm

The forearm is composed of the radius and the ulna. The radius is lateral to the ulna and follows the thumb upon pronation.

5. Wrist

The wrist is composed of two rows of four carpal bones (Fig.7-3). The most proximal row articulates with the radius

and ulna. It is composed of the *scaphoid, lunate, triquetrum* and *pisiform* from lateral to medial. The distal row is composed of the *trapezium, trapezoid, capitate* and *hamate*.

The scaphoid is boat-shaped. The middle third of this bone is narrowed and is called the *waist* of the scaphoid bone. On the lateral radiograph, the articular surface of the radius is normally tilted toward the palm of the hand (palmar tilt).

6. Hand

Digits of the hand are assigned numbers by convention to avoid confusion (Fig.7-3). Digit number one is the thumb

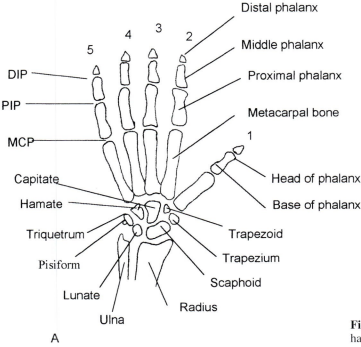

Distal phalanx
Middle phalanx
Proximal phalanx
Metacarpal bone
DIP
PIP
MCP
Capitate
Hamate
Triquetrum
Pisiform
Lunate
Ulna
Radius
Scaphoid
Trapezium
Trapezoid
Base of phalanx
Head of phalanx

A

Fig.7-3: **Hand and wrist anatomy.** A. Frontal view of the right hand. B. Lateral view of the right wrist.

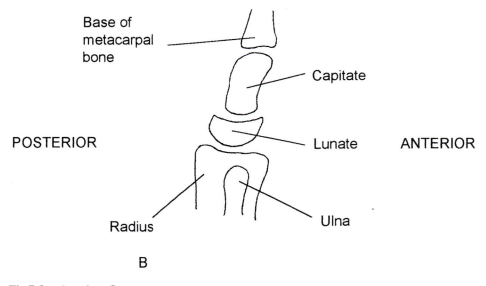

Fig.7-3: *(continued)*

(thumbs up for number one!). The small *pinky* finger is digit number five. Digits are composed of three phalanges, which are called proximal, middle and distal phalanges. The thumb, as an exception, lacks a middle phalanx and therefore is only composed of two phalanges. The phalangeal articulations are called the proximal interphalangeal (PIP) and the distal interphalangeal (DIP) joint. The 5 metacarpal bones make up the bulk of the hand. They articulate proximally with the carpal bones and distally with their respective digit at the metacarpophalangeal joint (MCP).

C. Lower limb

1. Hip

The femoral head articulates with the acetabulum of the pelvis much like a ball-in-socket. The femoral neck is located between the head and the greater and lesser trochanters (Fig.7-4).

Draw a line from the top of the greater trochanter to the top of the lesser trochanter. The capsule of the hip joint only extends down to this line. This fact is of major importance because the major blood supply (*circumflex arteries*) to the femoral head

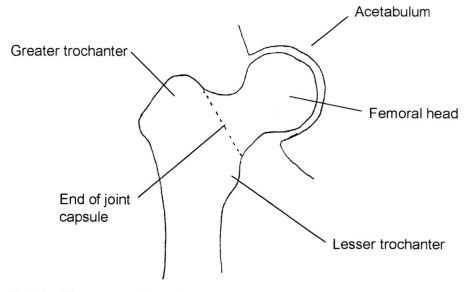

Fig.7-4: Hip anatomy. Frontal view.

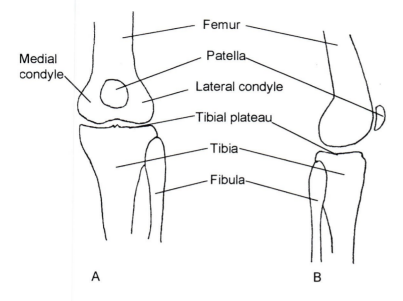

Fig.7-5: **Knee anatomy.** A. Frontal view. B. Lateral view.

comes via the capsule to this site to travel up to the femoral head. This means that any fracture between the trochanters (*intertrochanteric fracture*) and below this line will not interrupt the blood supply to the femoral head. However, any fracture above this line (*subcapital fracture*) will damage the femoral head blood supply and threaten femoral head viability.

2. Thigh (femoral shaft)

The femoral shaft is a tube-like structure.

3. Knee

The knee is composed of the medial and lateral condyles of the distal femur (Fig.7-5). These articulate with the top of

the tibia (*tibial plateau*). Note that the fibula does not participate in making the knee joint. The anterior distal femur also articulates with the patella.

4. Leg

The leg is composed of the tibia medially and the fibula laterally. The tibia is the major weight bearing bone of the leg.

5. Ankle

The distal tibia comprises two of the three *malleoli* (or bony bumps) of the ankle, which are the medial malleolus and the posterior malleolus (Fig.7-6). The remaining lateral malleolus arises from the fibula. The distal tibia and

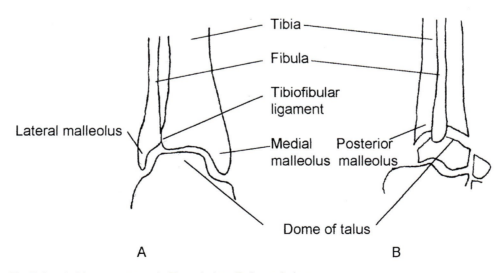

Fig.7-6: **Ankle anatomy.** A. Frontal view. B. Lateral view.

fibula are stabilized by the tibiofibular ligament. At the distal end of the tibia and fibula is the articular surface of the ankle, which rests on a dome shaped structure; the dome of the talus.

6. Foot

The foot is composed of several articulating tarsal bones. The heel is made of the calcaneus located just under the talus. These are followed by the *navicular,* the *cuboid* and the 3 *cuneiform* bones. More distally are 5 metatarsal bones, which articulate with their respective digits. As in the hand, the digits of the foot are assigned numbers, from 1 for the big toe to 5 for the small toe. The big toe is analogous to the thumb and has no middle phalanx. The proximal phalanges articulate with the metatarsal bones to make the metatarsophalangeal (MTP) joint. The articulation between two phalanges are either called a proximal interphalangeal (PIP) joint or a distal interphalangeal (DIP) joint depending on its location (Fig.7-7).

II. Approach

Often fractures can only be seen on one view. For this reason, one *must* always obtain two views of the bone being studied (AP and lateral).

1. Look for any abnormal black lines (fractures).
2. Look for any disruption of the cortex especially at the cortex lining the joints (intraarticular), which could represent a fracture. Remember that the cortex border should always be smooth.
3. *Look for any narrowing or widening of the joint space.*
4. *Look at the soft tissues for enlargement (swelling) or evidence of displaced fat pads (see section on radial head fracture).*

When a fracture is seen on a film, one *must* obtain films of the joint above and the joint below to rule out any associated fractures or dislocation.

Fracture description

It is common for students and interns to have to describe a fracture over the phone. The following terms are vital to do this:

> *Area.*   Area radiographed (i.e. Wrist)

> *Views.*   (i.e. AP and Lateral)

> *Location.*   Bone fractured. Part of the bone. Intraarticular or extraarticular (i.e. extraarticular distal radius fracture)

> *Pattern.*
- *Simple fracture:* The bone is broken in only two pieces. These are described by the direction of the fracture line (transverse, oblique, spiral, vertical).
- *Comminuted fracture:* The bone is broken in more than two pieces.
- *Compound fracture:* A fracture fragment extend through the skin or into an adjacent organ (i.e. the lung).

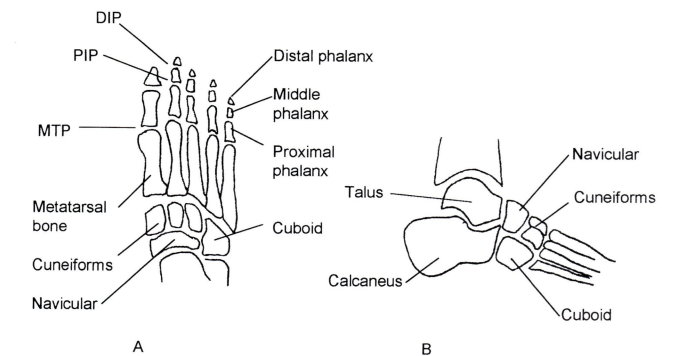

Fig.7-7:   Foot anatomy.   A. Frontal view. B. Lateral view.

Deformity (displacement)

- *Translation:* Decreased contact between the fracture surfaces (lateral, medial, anterior or posterior translation).
- *Angulation:* The bony fragments form an angle (apex lateral, apex medial, apex anterior and apex posterior).
- *Rotated:* The distal bony fragment is rotated in relation to the proximal one (external, internal rotation).
- *Impaction:* A bony fragment has been driven into an other.
- *Dislocation:* Misalignment of articulating surfaces of a joint (anterior or posterior dislocation).

Type

- *Pathologic fracture:* Fracture in an area of bone weakened by disease.
- *Stress fracture:* Fracture due to repetitive small traumas (i.e. marathon runner).

III. Specific problems

A. Upper Limb

1. Shoulder

a. Proximal humeral fracture

Proximal humeral fractures are classified depending on the number and amount of displacement of bony fragments seen *(Neer classification).* Proximal humeral fractures are associated with anterior and posterior dislocation of the glenohumeral joint (Fig.7-8). Proximal humeral fractures often occur in elderly patients after falling on an outstretched hand.

b. Glenohumeral joint dislocation

Anterior 90% of shoulder dislocations are anterior dislocations. The humeral head appears medial and inferior to the glenoid fossa on the frontal film (Fig.7-9A). On the trans-scapular view, there is disruption of the normal *Mercedes Benz* sign and the humeral head is displaced anteriorly (Fig.7-9B).

Commonly associated injuries with anterior shoulder dislocation are the *Hill-Sachs* lesion and the *Bankart* lesion (Fig.7-9C). A Hill-Sachs lesion is an impaction of the superolateral aspect of the humeral head against the glenoid caused by forceful contraction of shoulder muscle at the time the dislocation is taking place. The humeral head is left with a groove at the site of impact. Sometimes, the inferior glenoid rim is broken, which is called a Bankart lesion.

Posterior The humeral head appears superimposed on the glenoid and there is loss of the glenohumeral space on the frontal view (Fig.7-10A). On the trans-scapular

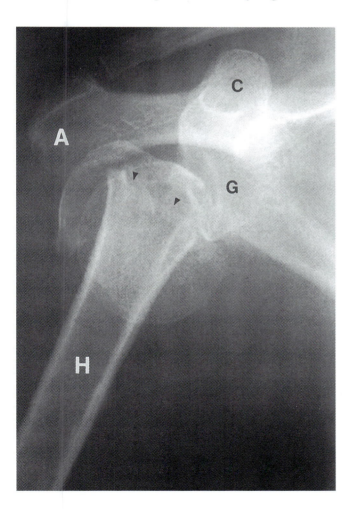

Fig.7-8: Proximal humeral fracture. Frontal shoulder radiograph showing a fracture (arrow heads) of the surgical neck of the right proximal humerus (H). Acromion (A). Glenoid (G). Coranoid (C).

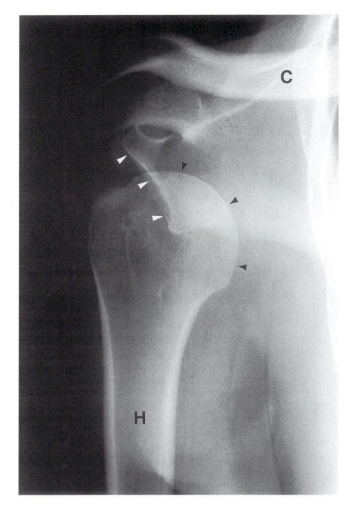

A

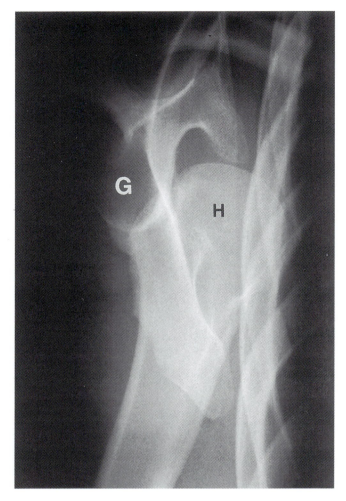

B

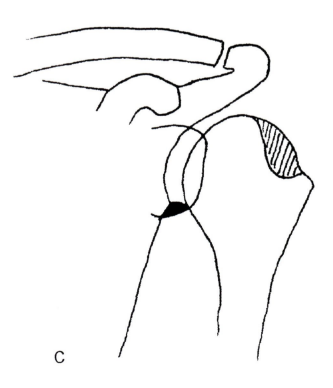

C

Fig.7-9:   Anterior shoulder dislocation.   A. Frontal radiograph of a left shoulder. The humeral head (black arrow heads) is medially and inferiorly displaced. It no longer articulates with glenoid fossa (white arrow heads). Humerus (H). Clavicle (C). B. Transscapular view showing anteroinferior displacement of the humeral head (H), which no longer articulates with the glenoid fossa (G). C. Frontal view showing the location of a Hill-Sachs lesion (lined area) and a Bankart lesion (black area).

view, the normal *Mercedes Benz* sign is again disrupted and the humeral head is located posterior to the glenoid (Fig.7-10B).

c. Acromioclavicular (AC) joint separation

AC separation is best seen on a clavicular view. Radiographs taken with the patient holding a small weight (i.e. 15 lbs) may also be obtained to make the diagnosis. There are three grades of AC separation (Fig.7-11). Grade one is when there is ligamentous injury without any abnormality seen on the radiograph. Grade two is when there is still some part of the clavicle associated with the acromion and grade three is when no association exists between the clavicle and the acromion. The mechanism of injury is falling on one's

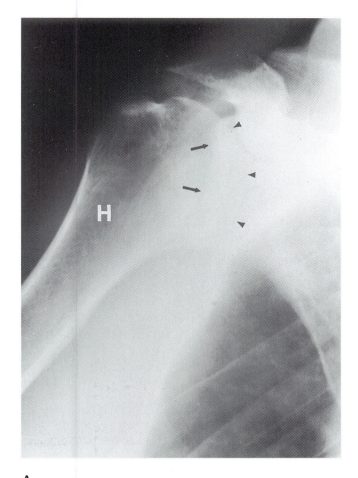

A

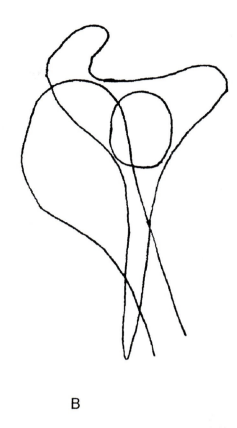

B

Fig.7-10: Posterior dislocation. A. Frontal radiograph of a shoulder showing overlap of the humeral head (arrow heads) and the glenoid fossa (arrows). B. Trans-scapular view showing posterior displacement of the humeral head.

shoulder much the way a football player would if tackled holding the football.

d. Clavicular fracture

Most clavicular fractures occur in the middle third of this bone. This is because the clavicle is S-shaped and is me-chanically weaker where it is curved. The mechanism of injury is the same as for AC separation.

2. Humeral shaft fracture

Humeral shaft fractures are commonly associated with radial nerve injury.

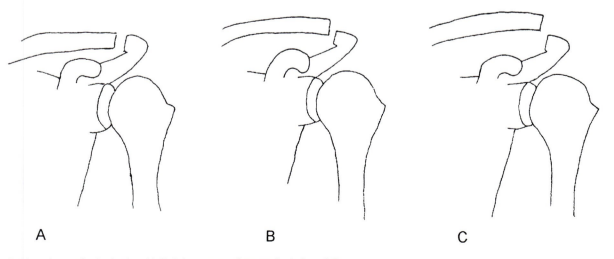

A   B   C

Fig.7-11: Acromioclavicular (AC) joint separation grade 1, 2 and 3.

3. Elbow

a. Distal humeral fracture

Distal humerus fractures are classified into three types (Fig.7-12):

1. *Supracondylar (extraarticular):* The fracture line is transverse above the condyles and does not involve the articular surface of the distal humerus.
2. *Transcondylar (intraarticular):* This fracture produces separation of either the lateral or medial condyle.
3. *Intercondylar (intraarticular):* This fracture is an injury which separates the two condyles.

b. Proximal ulnar fracture (olecranon fracture)

Olecranon fractures are usually intraarticular and are best seen on the lateral view of the elbow. The proximal fragment may be displaced because it is pulled by the triceps muscle. It is usually caused by a fall on a flexed elbow.

c. Elbow dislocation (+/− coronoid fracture)

The different types of elbow dislocation are classified by the relation of the ulna to the humerus. The most common type is by far the posterior dislocation of both the radius and the ulna (Fig.7-13). This injury is often associated with radial head and coronoid process fractures.

d. Radial head fracture

This fracture is usually intraarticular and may be difficult to see on standard views of the elbow. Two indirect signs may be seen due to elbow joint effusion, which displaces fat pads anterior and posterior to the distal humerus (Fig.7-14). These helpful signs in diagnosis of radial head fracture are called the *anterior* and *posterior fat pad signs.*

It is normal to see a small triangular shaped fat pad just anterior to the distal humerus (Fig.7-14A). This has the shape of the sail of a boat when there is no wind. When the anterior fat pad has the appearance of a sail on a windy day, there is a positive anterior fat pad sign (Fig.7-14BC). Normally, it is impossible to see the posterior fat pad (Fig. 7-14A). Any visualization of fat just posterior to the distal humerus is abnormal and constitutes a positive posterior fat pad sign (Fig.7-14BC).

4. Forearm

At an Italian student manifestation, the policeman Radii Galeazzi attempted to hit with a night stick one of the students called Ulna Monteggia. Ulna Monteggia blocked the blow with his forearm and proceded to trip Radii Galeazzi (the policeman), who fell on his outstretched hand. This story helps remember which bone is fractured and the mechanism of injury in *Galeazzi* and *Monteggia fracture-dislocation.*

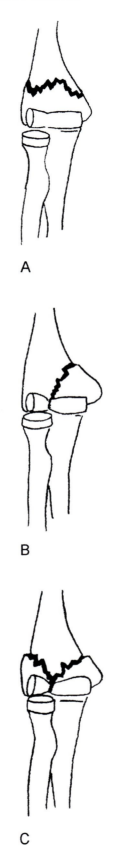

Fig.7-12: Distal humeral fractures. A. Supracondilar. B-Transcondylar. C. Intercondylar.

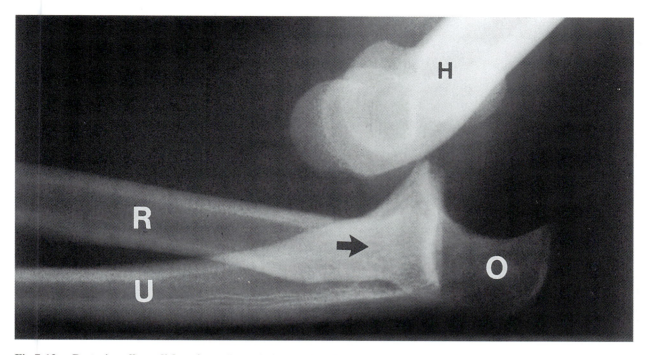

Fig.7-13: Posterior elbow dislocation. Lateral view of the elbow showing posterior displacement (black arrow) of the ulna (U) and the radius (R). Olecranon (O). Humerus (H).

a. Monteggia fracture dislocation (night-stick injury)

A Monteggia fracture-dislocation is a fracture of the ulna with associated dislocation of the radial head at the elbow (Fig.7-15). It is usually caused by receiving a blow on the forearm when one is trying to protect oneself (Just like the student Ulna Monteggia in the story).

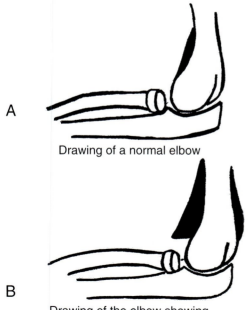

A

Drawing of a normal elbow

B

Drawing of the elbow showing positive anterior and posterior fat pad signs

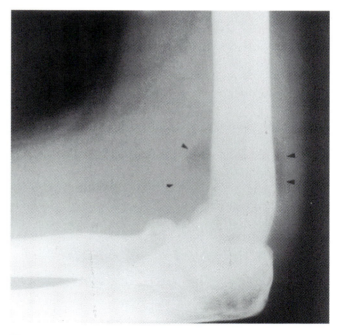

C

Fig.7-14: Radial head fracture. A. Drawing of a normal elbow. No posterior fat pad and only a small anterior fat pad is seen. B. Drawing of the elbow showing positive anterior and posterior fat pad signs. C. Lateral radiograph of the elbow showing positive anterior and posterior fat pad signs (arrow head).

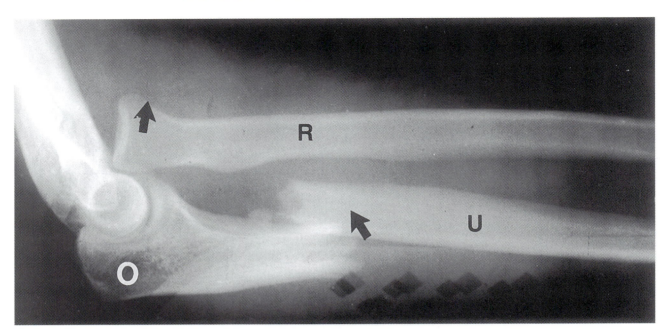

Fig.7-15: Monteggia fracture dislocation. Lateral radiograph of the forearm showing fracture (arrow) of the ulna (U) and proximal dislocation (arrow) of the radius (R). Olecranon (O).

b. Galeazzi fracture-dislocation

A Galeazzi fracture dislocation is a fracture of the distal radius with associated dislocation of the distal radio-ulnar joint at the wrist (Fig.7-16). The mechanism of injury is a fall on an outstretched hand (just like the policeman Radii Galeazzi in the story).

5. Wrist

a. Colles' fracture

This injury is an extraarticular fracture of the distal radius with dorsal displacement of the distal fragment with the apex palmar angulation (Fig.7-17A). On the lateral radiograph, the wrist takes on the appearance of a dinner fork (*dinner fork deformity*). The distal fragment is often impacted into the proximal one which gives rise to shortening of the radius. Half of patients with a Colle's fracture also have a fracture of the ulnar styloid. This injury is often caused by falling on an outstretched hand.

b. Smith's fracture

Smith's fractures are either extra or intraarticular. These fractures are essentially inverted Colle's fracture since there is apex dorsal angulation (Fig.7-17B). If the fracture is intraarticular, it is called a *Barton's fracture*.

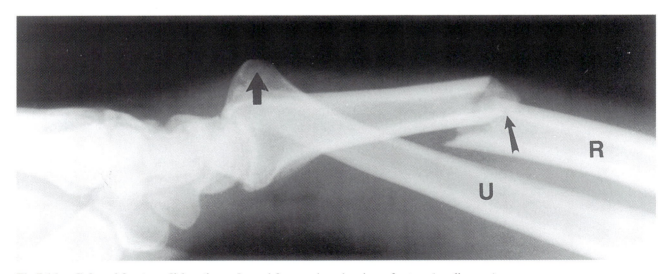

Fig.7-16: Galeazzi fracture dislocation. Lateral forearm view showing a fracture (small arrow) of the radius (R). The distal ulna (U) is dislocated (thick arrow) dorsally.

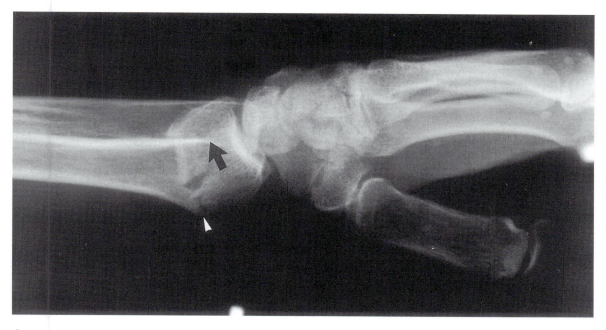

A

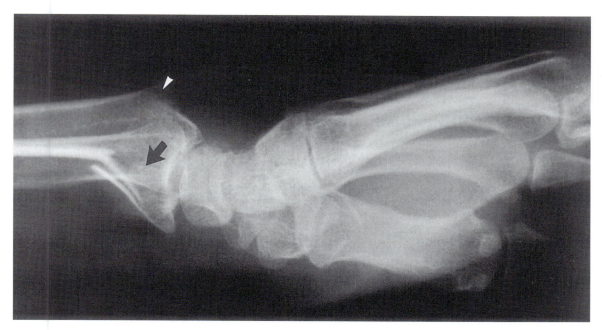

B

Fig.7-17: Distal radial fractures. A. Colles' fracture. Lateral radiograph of the wrist showing a distal radial fracture (white arrow head). The distal fragment is posteriorly displaced (black arrow). B. Smith's fracture. Lateral radiograph of the wrist showing a distal radial fracture (white arrow head) with anterior displacement of the distal fragment (black arrow).

c. Scaphoid fracture

The boat-shaped scaphoid bone is the most commonly fractured carpal bone. It usually breaks at its waist (Fig.7-18). Because the only blood supply to this bone is distal to proximal, the fracture may interrupt the feeding vessels to the proximal portion of the bone, which can give rise to bone death (*avascular necrosis*).

d. Wrist dislocations

Carpal dislocations are best visualized on a lateral radiograph of the wrist.

Perilunate dislocation This injury is a dorsal dislocation of the capitate bone. The lunate bone is still aligned with the radius (Fig.7-19).

Lunate dislocation   This injury is a palmar dislocation of the lunate bone. The capitate remains aligned with the radius.

6. Hand

a. First metacarpal base fractures

Once, the great singer Tony Bennett was being driven by his chauffeur Rolando. Suddenly the engine broke and they had to hitch-hike for hours. Although both of them had sore thumbs, Rolando's thumb hurt the most because he did most of the hitch-hiking. This story helps remember that *Bennett's* and *Rolando's fractures* are located at the first metacarpal base and that Rolando's fracture is the worse.

Bennett's fracture   A Bennett's fracture is a single intraarticular fracture of the base of the first metacarpal bone (Fig.7-20A). The large distal fragment is dislocated radially and

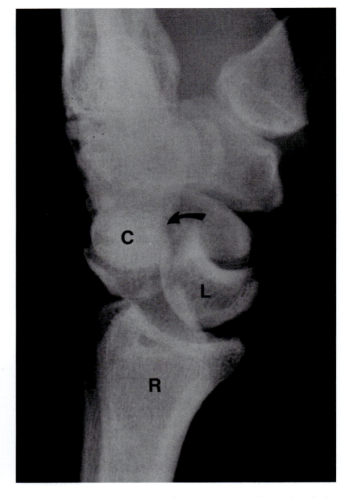

Fig.7-19: Perilunate dislocation. Lateral radiograph of the wrist showing dorsal dislocation (arrow) of the capitate bone (C). The lunate bone (L) is still aligned with the radius (R).

dorsally by the *abductor pollicis longus* muscle. Bennett's fracture must be distinguished from extraarticular fractures of the same site because it usually requires an open reduction.

Rolando's fracture   The Rolando fracture (Fig.7-20B) is a comminuted Bennett's fracture and requires open reduction and internal fixation.

b. Skier's thumb (Gamekeeper's thumb)

The Skier's thumb is a fracture of the base of the proximal phalanx of the thumb (Fig.7-20C) with disruption of the ulnar collateral ligament. This entity is common in down hill skiing when one's thumb is stressed by getting trapped in a ski pole.

c. Boxer's fracture

The boxer's fracture is a fracture of the fifth metacarpal neck with apex dorsal angulation and external rotation of the

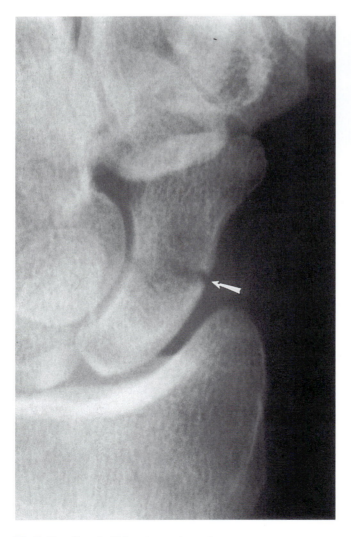

Fig.7-18: Scaphoid fracture   (arrow).

distal fragment (Fig.7-20D). It is usually caused by punching a hard surface like a wall.

d. Baseball (Mallet) finger

The baseball finger is usually caused by a hyperflexion injury at the DIP joint (Fig.7-20E). This results in avulsion of the extensor tendon with or without associated avulsion fracture of the proximal dorsal aspect of the distal phalanx. It is often caused by receiving a projectile such as a baseball on ones finger tip.

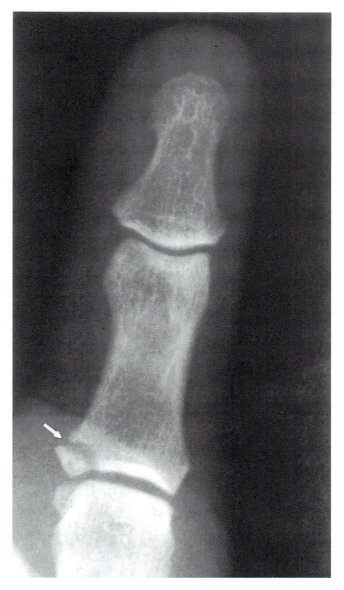

C

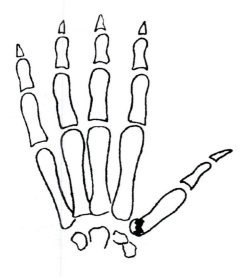

A

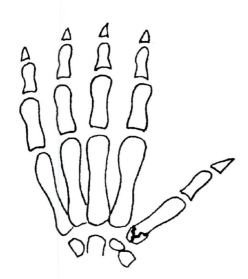

B

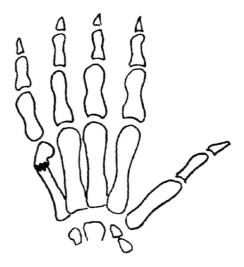

D

Fig.7-20:   Hand fractures.   A. Bennett's fracture. B. Rolando's fracture. C. Skier's thumb. D. Boxer's fracture. E. Baseball finger.

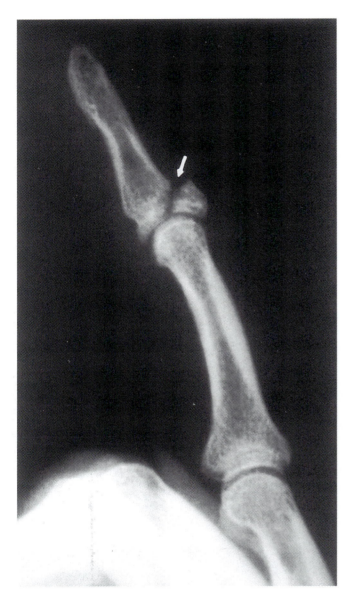

E

Fig.7-20 (*continued*)

B. Lower limb

1. Hip

a. Hip fractures

Subcapital A subcapital fracture is just under the caput or head of the femur (Fig.7-21A). It is common and frequently gives rise to avascular necrosis (bone death).

Intertrochanteric An Intertrochanteric fracture joins the greater and lesser trochanters (Fig.7-21B). It is less common than a subcapital fracture, and. avascular necrosis is infrequent.

Subtrochanteric A subtrochanteric fracture is a transverse, spiral or oblique fracture of the proximal femur that is located below the lesser trochanter.

b. Hip dislocations

Posterior 90% of hip dislocations are posterior. In this injury, the femoral head is also displaced superiolaterally in relation to the acetabulum (Fig.7-22A). It is often associated with posterior acetabular rim frac-

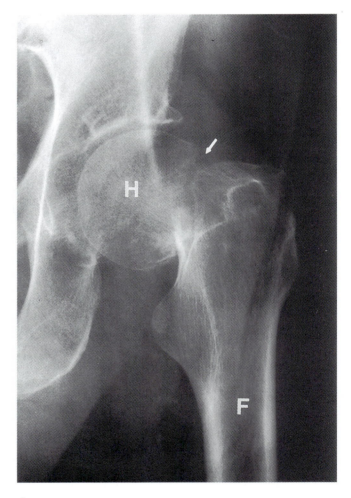

A

Fig.7-21: Hip fractures. A. Frontal radiograph of the left hip showing a subcapital fracture (arrow). B. Frontal radiograph of the left hip showing an intertrochanteric fracture (arrows). Femur (F). Femoral head (H).

tures. The mechanism of injury is an impact on the knee with the hip flexed (e.g. hitting the dashboard in a motor vehicle accident).

Anterior In anterior dislocation of the hip, the femoral head is also displaced inferomedially in relation to the acetabulum (Fig.7-22B). It is the result of a forced hip abduction.

2. Femoral shaft fracture

Femoral shaft fractures are the result of a significant impact and are often of the spiral pattern.

3. Knee

a. Tibial plateau fracture

Tibial plateau fractures can be simple, comminuted or depressed. Since it is most common to be hit at the lateral as-

pect of the knee, it is not surprising that the lateral tibial plateau is most often fractured (Fig.7-23).

b. Patellar fracture

The patella is most frequently fractured transversely, although vertical or comminuted fractures are also sometimes seen (Fig.7-24). Be aware that a normal patella may be in multiple parts (*multipartite patella*). The fact that the pieces of bone do not fit together well and that the edges are well corticated helps differentiate it from a fracture.

4. Tibial and fibular fractures

Tibial and fibular shaft fractures are common and are usually of a spiral pattern.

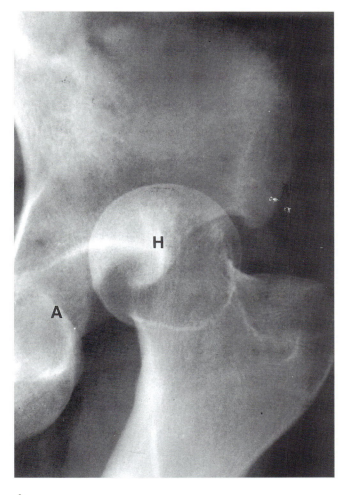

A

Fig.7-22: Hip dislocations. A. Posterior hip dislocation. Frontal radiograph of the left hip showing superolateral displacement of femoral head (H). It no longer articulates with the acetabulum (A). B. Anterior hip dislocation. Frontal view of the left hip showing inferomedial displacement of the femoral head (H). It no longer articulates with the acetabulum (A).

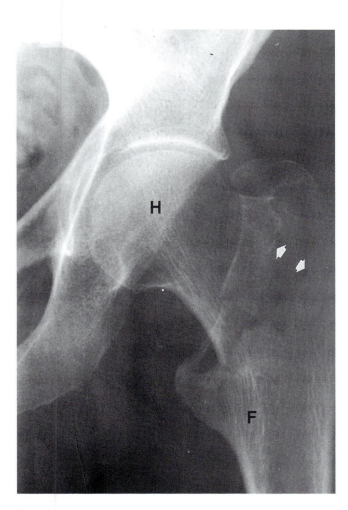

B

Fig.7-21 (*continued*)

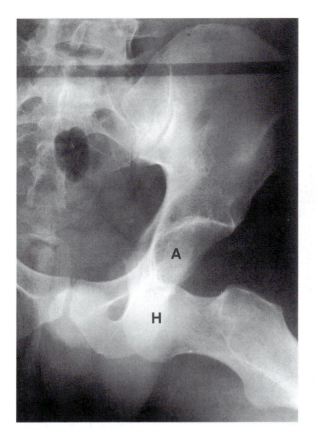

B

Fig.7-22 (*continued*)

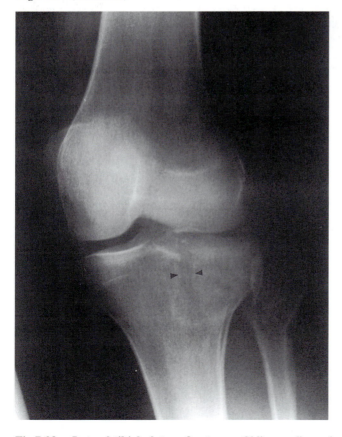

Fig.7-23: Lateral tibial plateau fracture. Oblique radiograph of the left knee showing a lateral tibial plateau fracture (arrow head).

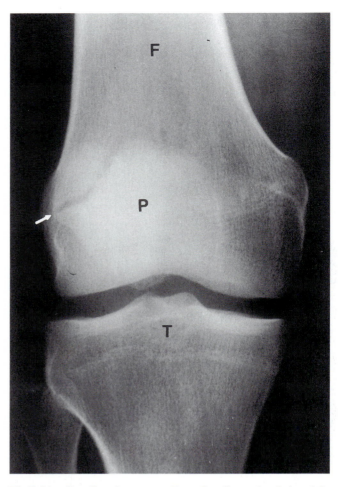

Fig.7-24: Patellar fracture. Frontal radiograph of the right knee showing a fracture (arrow) in the patella (P). Femur (F). Tibia (T).

5. Ankle fracture

When evaluating ankle radiographs for fractures, first ensure that all three malleoli are intact (Fig.7-25).The joint space between the distal tibia and the dome of the talus (*mortice*) should be even throughout.

A simple ankle fracture classification includes type A, B, and C. In type A , the fracture occurs below the tibiofibular ligament ,while B is through the ligament and C is above. All three types include medial malleolar fractures (tibial side). The single medial maleolus fracture is often associated with a proximal fibular fracture (*Maisonneuve fracture*).

6. Foot

a. Calcaneal (lover's) fracture

It is often difficult to see the fracture line in a calcaneal fracture. Measure *Boehler's angle* as shown (Fig.7-26). An angle of less than 28 degree indicates that there is a fracture of the calcaneus. This injury is caused by a fall from height much like a lover jumping from a balcony in order to avoid an encounter with a furious husband.

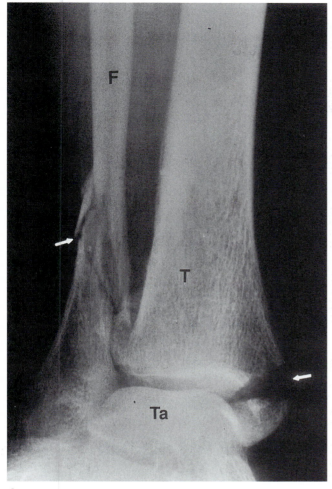

A

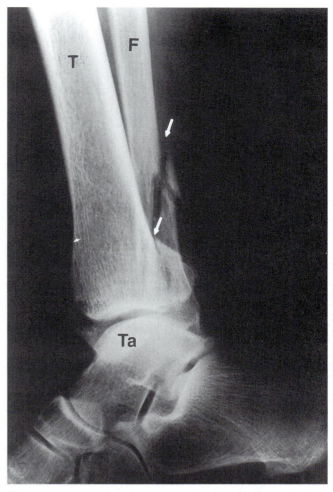

B

Fig.7-25: Trimalleolar ankle fracture. A. Frontal radiograph of the right ankle showing fractures (arrows) of the lateral and medial malleolus. B. Lateral radiograph of the ankle showing posterior malleolus and fibular fractures (arrows). Fibula (F). Tibia (T). Talus (Ta).

Calcaneal fractures are often associated with thoracolumbar burst fractures (see Axial Skeleton chapter) and ankle fractures. Therefore one *must* obtain views of the thoracolumbar spine if a calcaneal fracture is found.

b. March fracture

A march fracture is a stress fracture of the second or third metatarsal bone (Fig.7-27) caused by repetitive minor trauma such as when an army recruit marches excessively.

c. Jones' fracture

A Jones' fracture is a stress fracture of the base of the fifth metatarsal (Fig.7-28). It more common in athletes.

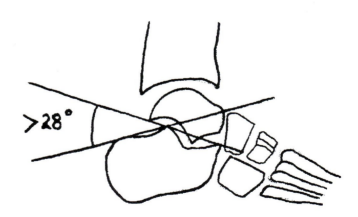

A

Fig.7-26: Calcaneal fracture. A. Boehler's angle. Boehler's angle is normally more than 28 degrees. B. Calcaneal fracture. Lateral view of the foot showing a fracture (arrow heads) extending to the talocalcaneal joint (white arrow). Boehler's angle is 15 degrees.

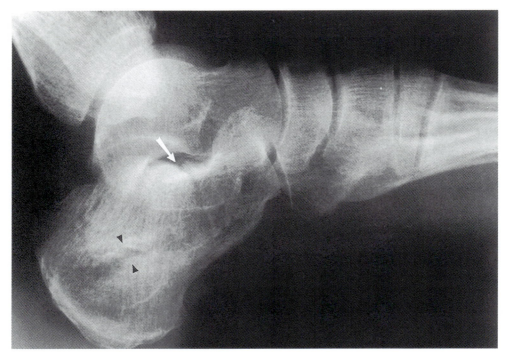

B

Fig.7-26 (*continued*)

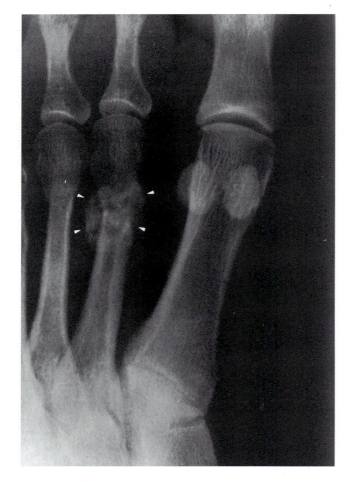

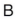

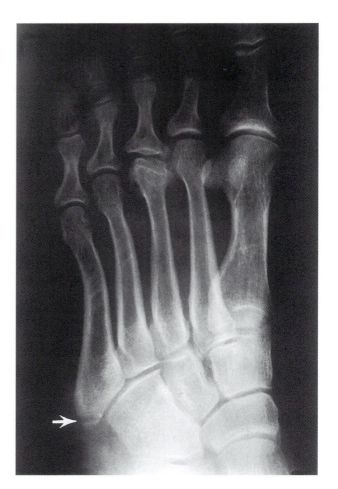

Fig.7-27: **March fracture.** Magnified frontal radiograph of the left foot showing a fracture with callus formation (arrow heads) of the diaphysis of the second metatarsal bone.

Fig.7-28: **Jones' fracture.** Frontal radiograph of the foot showing a fracture (arrow) of the base of the 5th metatarsal bone.

Chapter 8.   Non-Traumatic Skeletal Radiology

I. Infection

A. Osteomyelitis

In osteomyelitis, an infection destroys bone (*lytic lesion*). Sometimes a devascularized piece of bone (*sequestrum*) may persist in the lesion. Adjacent periosteum may get inflamed and thickened (*periostitis*). The infection may also extend to adjacent joints (*septic arthritis*) or intervertebral disk (*diskitis*). Osteomyelitis is common and may occur in any patient of any age.

On the radiograph, look for (Fig.8-1):

1. *Lytic lesion* (dark focal area)
2. *Sequestrum* (bright spot in the lytic lesion)
3. *Periostitis* (Soft tissue strip along the bone)

Remember that the radiograph may be normal in the first 10 days of infection.

B. Septic arthritis

In septic arthritis, infection gives rise to joint effusion and swelling of adjacent soft tissue. The bone on each side of the joint may become demineralized (focal *osteopenia*). Eventually, there may be destruction of articular cartilage.

On the radiograph, look for (Fig.8-2):

1. *Soft tissue swelling* (enlarged soft tissue)
2. *Periarticular osteopenia* (dark area on each side of the joint)
3. *Joint space narrowing* (thinner joint line because of cartilage destruction)

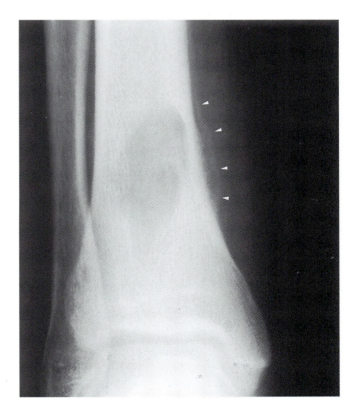

A

Fig.8-1: Osteomyelitis (i.e. Brodie's abscess). A. Magnified radiograph of the right ankle showing a large lytic tibial lesion. Notice the periosteal reaction medial to the tibia (arrow heads). B. Radiograph of the distal femur showing a large lytic lesion containing a sequestrum (arrow head).

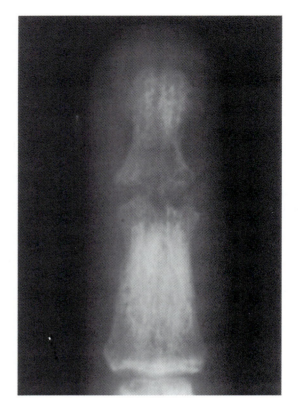

A

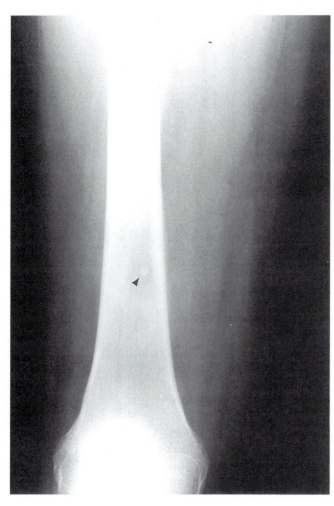

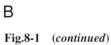

B

Fig.8-1   (continued)

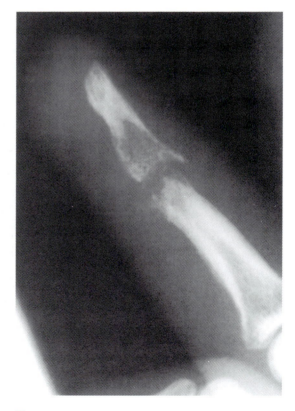

B

Fig.8-2: Septic arthritis.   Magnified radiograph of the DIP joint of the 2nd digit showing joint space narrowing, periarticular osteopenia and soft tissue swelling. A-Frontal radiograph B. Lateral radiograph.

II. Osteoarthritis

Osteoarthitis (OA) is caused by wear and tear of articular cartilage. It is often seen in weight bearing joints, such as the knees, the hips and the spine. DIP and PIP joints are also often involved. Ultimately, bone rubs against bone and causes an inflammatory reaction, swelling and pain. Often the bone near the joint reacts to form bony spurs (*osteophytes*). Sometimes areas of bony degeneration form cysts in the subarticular bone (*subarticular cysts*).

On the radiograph, look for (Fig.8-3):

1. *Asymmetric joint space narrowing*
2. *Periarticular sclerosis* (whiter than normal area on each side of the bone)
3. *Osteophytes*
4. *Subarticular cysts* (black round spots)

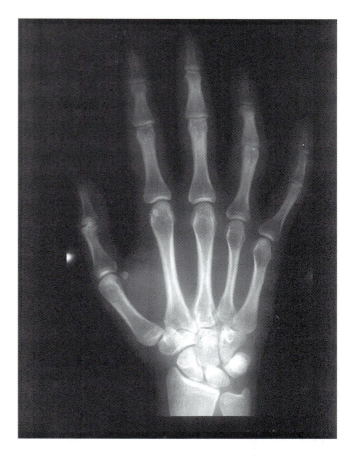

A

Fig.8-3: Osteoarthritis (OA). A. Radiograph of normal right hand. B. Extensive OA of the hands. C. Radiograph of a normal right hip. D. Magnified radiograph of the right hip showing periarticular sclerosis (black arrow heads) and osteophytes (white arrow). Notice also the joint space narrowing especially superiorly.

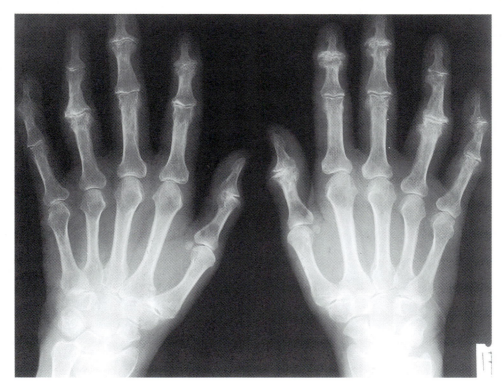

B

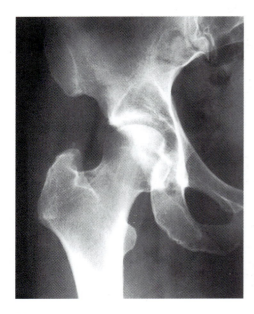

C

Fig.8-3   (*continued*)

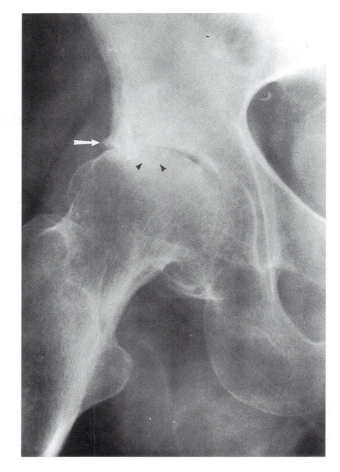

D

III. Inflammation

A. Rheumatoid arthritis

Rheumatoid arthritis (RA) is an inflammatory process of the synovium. It results in soft tissue swelling, articular cartilage destruction, periarticular demineralization and bony erosion. It is usually symmetrical. RA is more frequent in females.

On the radiograph, look for (Fig.8-4):

1. *Soft tissue swelling*
2. *Periarticular osteopenia*
3. *Bony erosion*
4. *Joint subluxation*
5. *No osteophytes*

B. Ankylosing spondylitis

Ankylosing Spondylitis (AS) is an inflammatory process, which causes sclerosis and fusion of the SI joints (*sacroiliitis*). The vertebrae become bridged by ligamentous calcifications (*syndesmophytes*), which gives a bamboo stick appearance to the spine (Fig.8-5).

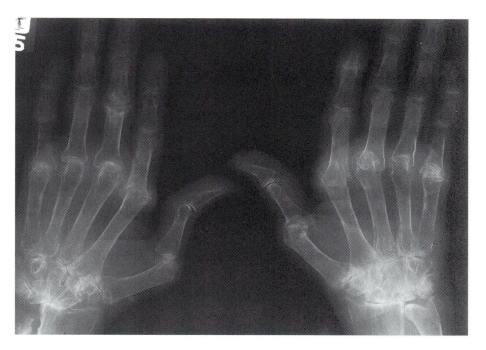

Fig.8-4: Rheumatoid arthritis (RA). Frontal radiograph of the hands showing periarticular osteopenia, bony erosions and MCP joint subluxation. Notice the absence of osteophytes.

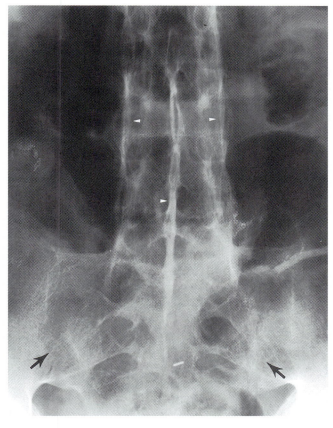

A

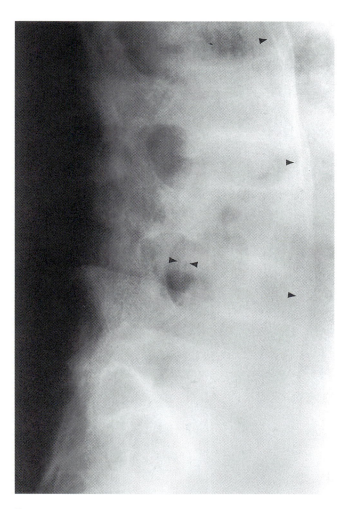

B

Fig.8-5: Ankylosing spondylitis (AS). A. Frontal radiograph of the lumbar spine. B. Lateral radiograph of the lumbar spine. Notice the blurred SI joints (arrows) secondary to sacroilitis. There are also syndesmophytes (arrow heads) giving the spine a bamboo appearance.

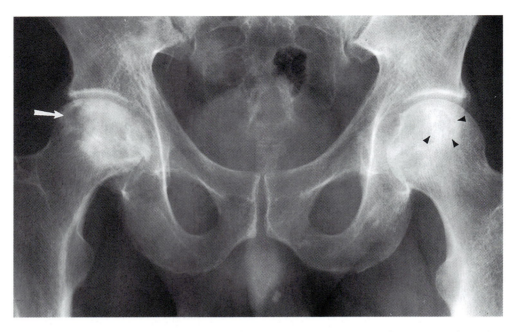

Fig.8-6:   Bilateral hip avascular necrosis (AVN).   Magnified radiograph of the hips showing collapse (white arrow) and sclerosis of the right femoral head. The left femoral head exhibits some sclerosis (black arrow heads).

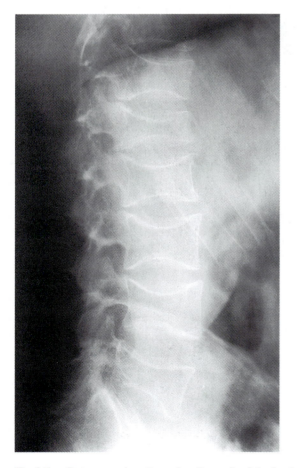

Fig.8-7:   Osteoporosis.   Lateral radiograph of the lumbar spine showing typical collapse of all the vertebral bodies. The vertebral bodies are biconcave instead of the normal square shape.

IV. Avascular necrosis

Avascular necrosis (AVN) is bone death cause by poor blood supply to an area of bone. For example, AVN often occurs in the femoral head.

On the radiograph, look for (Fig.8-6):

1. *Osteopenia* (low bone density)
2. *Sclerosis*
3. *Dark crescent* (femoral head)
4. *Collapse*

Remember that AVN only affects one side of the articulation (i.e. femoral head). It does not affect the other side of the joint (i.e. acetabulum) since it has a different blood supply.

V. Metabolic

A. Osteoporosis

Osteoporosis is a state of diffuse low bone density (darker than normal) often caused by old age or postmenopausal state. In other words, there is a decreased amount of normal bone. This often results in pathological fractures. In the spine, osteoporosis gives rise to typical biconcave collapse of the vertebral bodies (Fig.8-7).

B. Paget's disease

Paget's disease usually starts after the fourth decade of life. There is bone destruction (*lytic phase*) followed by deposition of thick weak bone (*sclerotic phase*). Therefore, long bones often bow or fracture. Paget's disease involves the pelvis, the femur and the skull most frequently (Fig.8-8).

VI. Tumors

Bone tumors are usually lytic lesions (darker than normal). Remember that some tumors such as breast and prostate metastasis to the bone can be sclerotic (whiter than normal).

A. Malignant

Malignant bone tumors have a more aggressive pattern of bone destruction. On the radiograph, look for a wide area of transition between the lesion and normal bone. Also look for cortical destruction, periosteal reaction and soft tissue mass (Fig.8-9A).

B. Benign

Benign bone tumors have less aggressive pattern of bone destruction. On the radiograph, look for a sharp area of transition between the lesion and normal bone. There should be no cortical destruction (Fig.8-9B).

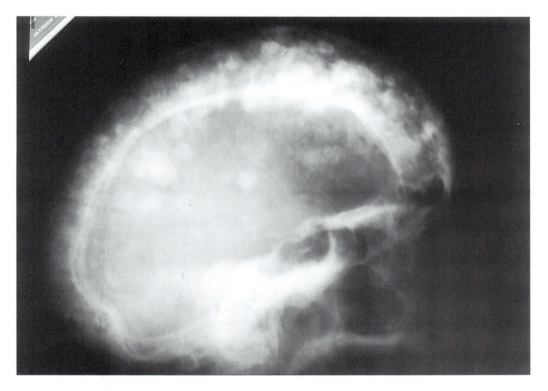

A

Fig.8-8:   Paget's disease.   A. Lateral radiograph of the skull showing gross widening of the skull thickness and extensive patchy sclerosis. B. frontal view of the pelvis showing thickening of bony structures with lytic-sclerotic changes. C. Frontal radiograph of the right hip showing bone thickening and bowing of the femur. Notice the small fractures (arrow heads) in the femoral shaft.

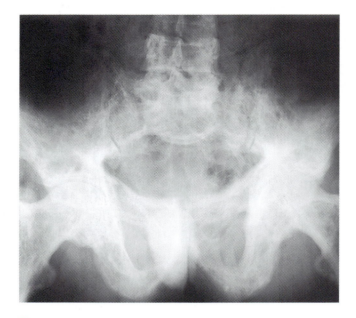

B

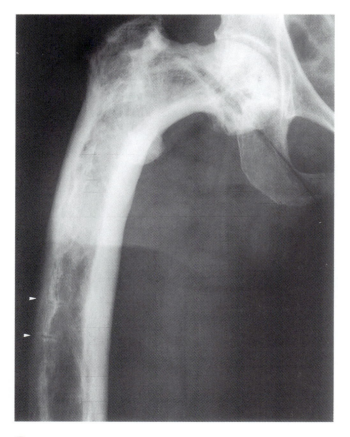

C

Fig.8-8   (*continued*)

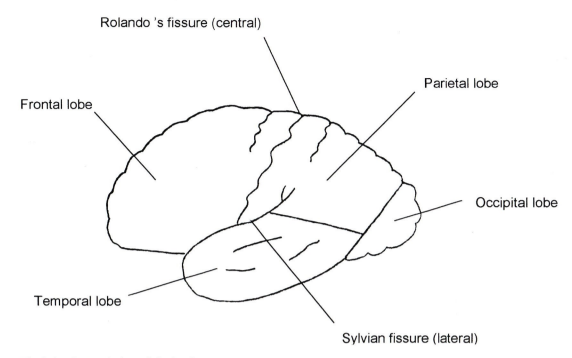

Fig.9-1: Lateral view of the brain.

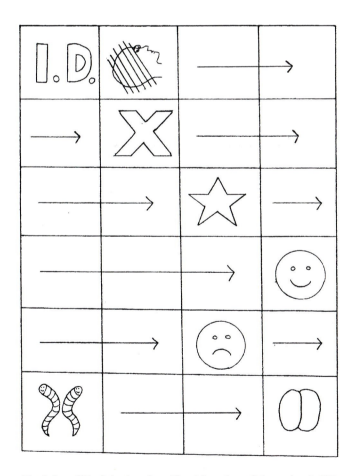

Fig.9-2: CT of the head: Usual location of the patient's I.D., Scout view, and the 6 essential CT images. The other boxes represent images taken between the essential images.

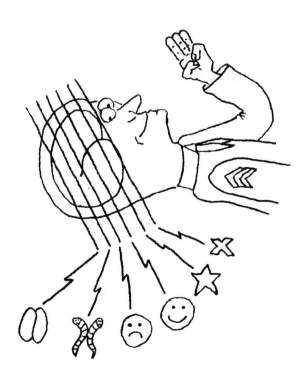

Fig.9-3: Scout view. Magnified view of the 2nd box, 1st row of fig.9-2. The Scout view of a CT scan looks like a plain radiograph of the patient in profile. 6 lines are drawn on the diagram to indicate the levels at which the 6 essential CT images are taken.

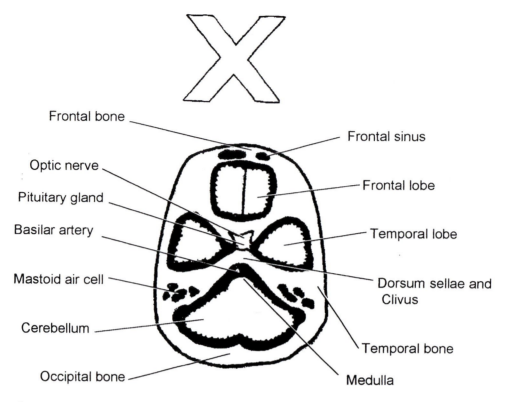

Frontal bone

Frontal sinus

Optic nerve

Pituitary gland

Frontal lobe

Basilar artery

Temporal lobe

Mastoid air cell

Dorsum sellae and Clivus

Cerebellum

Temporal bone

Occipital bone

Medulla

A

Fig.9-4:   The X.   1st basic slice taken near the base of the skull.
A. Diagram of normal anatomy. B. CT image of normal anatomy.
C. MRI of the author's head (Hopefully normal).

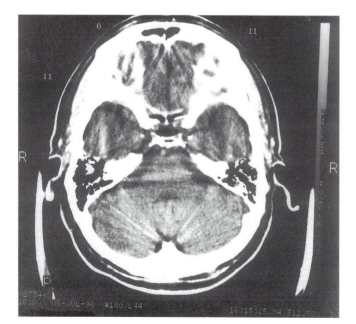

B

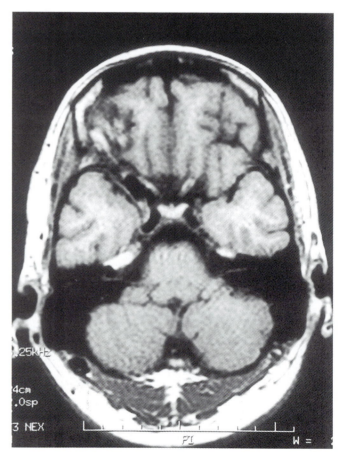

C

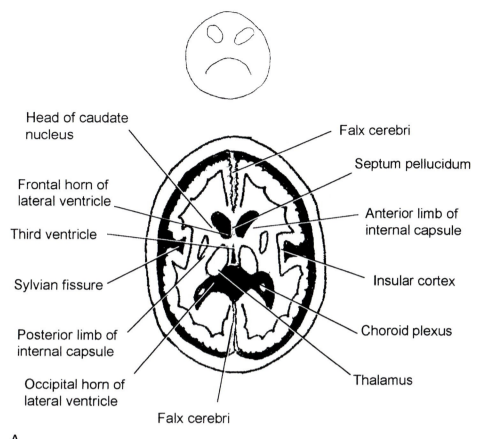

Head of caudate nucleus

Falx cerebri

Septum pellucidum

Frontal horn of lateral ventricle

Third ventricle

Anterior limb of internal capsule

Sylvian fissure

Insular cortex

Posterior limb of internal capsule

Choroid plexus

Occipital horn of lateral ventricle

Thalamus

Falx cerebri

A

Fig.9-7: **Mr. Sad** 4th basic slice. A. Diagram of normal anatomy. B. CT image of normal anatomy. C. MRI of the author's head.

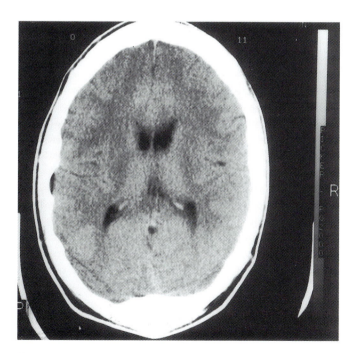

B

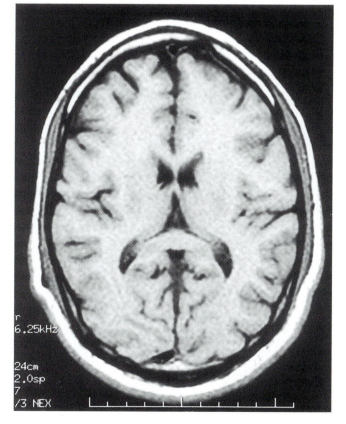

C

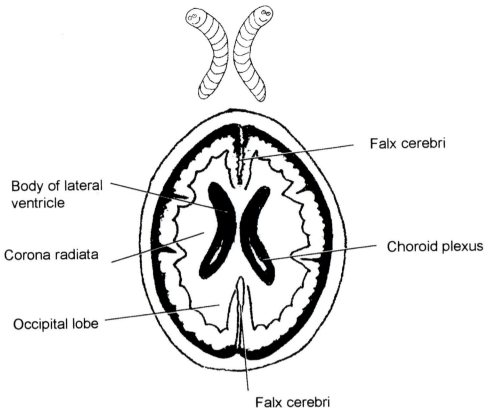

Falx cerebri

Body of lateral ventricle

Corona radiata

Occipital lobe

Choroid plexus

Falx cerebri

A

Fig.9-8: The Worms 5th basic slice. A. Diagram of normal anatomy. B. CT image of normal anatomy. C. MRI image of the author's head.

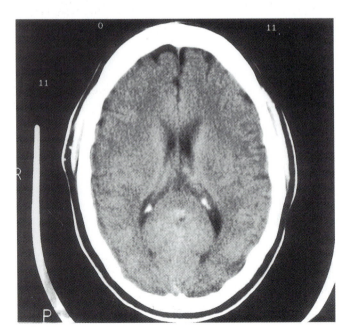

B

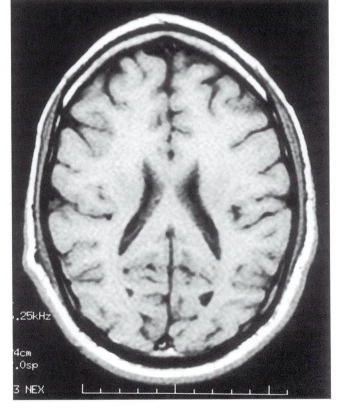

C

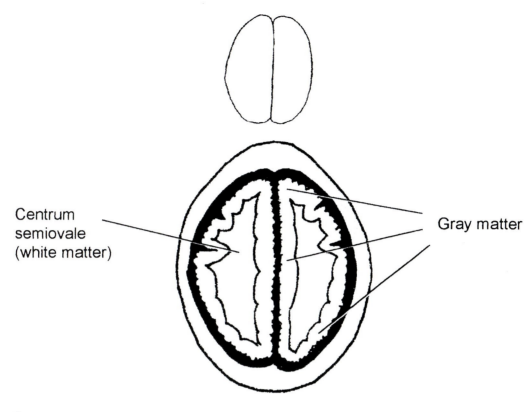

A

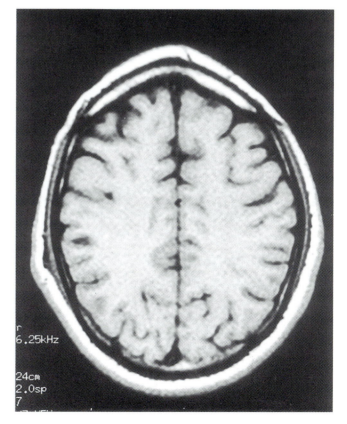

Fig.9-9: **The Coffee Bean** 6th basic slice. A. diagram of normal anatomy. B. CT image of normal anatomy. C. MRI image of the author's head.

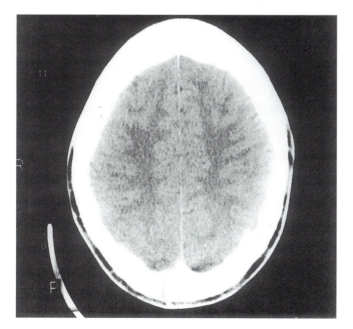

B

C

anterior, middle, and posterior part of the brain from the "X" to "Mr. Sad" level (Fig.9-10A). However, from the "Worm" to the "Coffee Bean" level, the anterior cerebral artery supplies most of the midline from anterior to posterior (Fig.9-10B).

C. Ventricular system

The ventricular system contains the *cerebrospinal fluid* (*CSF*) and is composed of the lateral ventricles, the *foramina of Monro,* the third ventricle, the *aqueduct of Sylvius,*

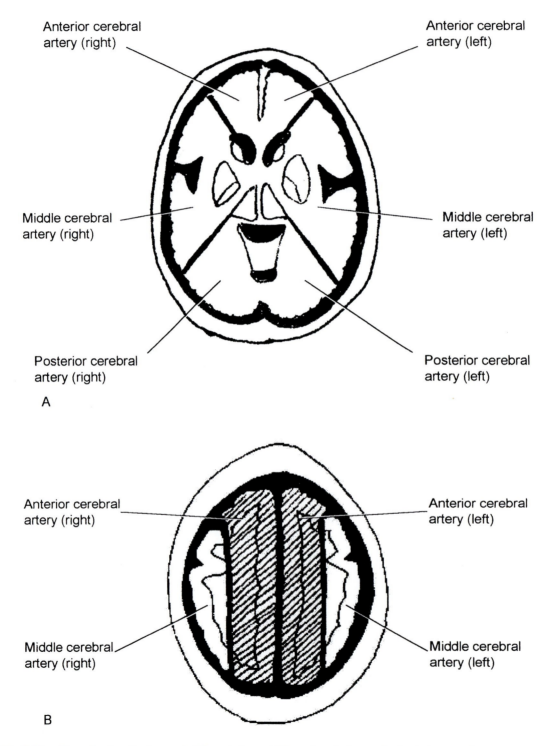

Fig.9-10: Vascular territories. A. The anterior, middle and posterior cerebral arteries grossly supply the anterior, middle and posterior part of the brain from the *X* to the *Mr. Sad* levels. B. From the *Worms* to the *Coffee Bean* level, the anterior cerebral arteries supply most of the midline.

and the fourth ventricle. All of these structures are interconnected (Fig.9-11). The *choroid plexi* located throughout this system make CSF. The CSF flows down the ventricles and exits through the *foramina of Magendie* and *Lushka* to reach the *subarachnoid spaces* (cistern and space around the brain). CSF is then resorbed through the *arachnoid granulation tissue* on top of the brain, into a big vein, called the *superior sagittal sinus.*

II. Approach

To remember the approach to CT (*CAT*) scans of the *head,* remember the story of the showbiz *cat* who was trying to get a*head:* Once a cat called *X* easily recognized by his *black* and *white* spots was a *ventriloquist.* One day, he had his big *break* and *masses* came to see him (Fig.9-12).

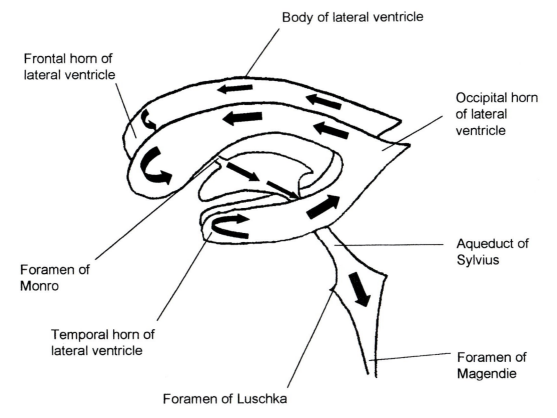

Fig.9-11: Ventricular system anatomy. Large black arrows indicate the direction of CSF flow.

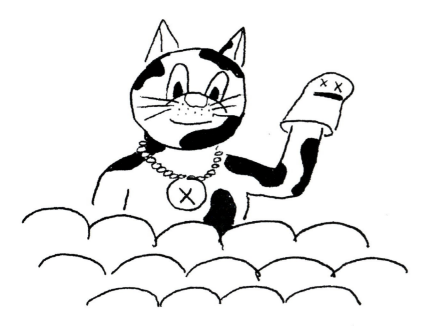

Fig.9-12: Showbiz cat. To remember the approach to CAT scans of the head, remember the showbiz cat that was trying to get ahead.

1. The *X*

Look at the "X" level. Specifically look at the lower leg of the "X" itself, which represents the mastoid air cells, to see if they are of the same thickness on both sides. This is to determine if the slices were taken at the same level on each side. If the patient's head had been tilted in the CT scanner, these structures will appear asymmetrical. This may account for apparent asymmetry between the cerebral hemispheres or other structures on several or all images.

2. *Black* Strokes

Look for any abnormally black (dark) area, which could represent an infarcted portion of brain (discussed in Stroke section).

3. *White* Hemorrhage

Look for any abnormally white (bright) area, which could represent acute hemorrhage in the ventricular system, in the brain, or around it (discussed in Hemorrhage section).

4. *Ventriloquist* Ventricular and sulcal size

Look at the ventricles to see if they are abnormally enlarged. Look at the sulci to see if they are too big or too small (discussed in Hydrocephalus section)

5. *Break* Fractures

Look for abnormal dark lines in the white bone (fractures) and for black air inside the skull (discussed in Trauma section).

6. *Mass* and/or Mass effect

Look for any big mass (tumor or abscess) in the brain. Ensure that the brain is not pushed to one side because of a mass or intracranial hemorrhage.

III. Specific problems

A. Hemorrhage

The CT appearance of fresh blood (also known as acute hemorrhage) is that of a white (*hyperdense*) area in comparison to the gray colored brain. After a week, blood starts to appear gray like the brain or slightly darker than the brain. At this point, it is called a subacute hemorrhage (*isodense* or slightly *hypodense*). After several weeks, blood appears much darker than the gray brain, and it is then called a chronic hemorrhage (*hypodense*). Bleeds may occur in four areas within the skull, as intraparenchymal, subarachnoid, subdural or epidural hemorrhages.

1. Intraparenchymal

Acute intraparenchymal hemorrhage is easily recognized on CT scans as an abnormal white area in the brain tissue. As the blood becomes older, it degrades and eventually becomes darker than brain tissue (chronic). Intraparenchymal hemorrhage is bleeding within the brain tissue itself. It is most commonly caused by hypertension, but is also seen with trauma, brain malignancy or infarct (see section on hemorrhagic stroke).

2. Subarachnoid

On CT scan, some of the CSF appears white rather than its usual dark appearance, because it is mixed with bright blood. Hemorrhage is seen in the Sylvian fissure, the suprasellar cistern (Fig.9-13), the basal cistern and the quadrigeminal cistern (Fig.9-6). There may also be bright blood in the ventricles. The best location to examine for intraventricular hemorrhage is the occipital horns of the lateral ventricles, where the blood collects due to gravity (Fig.9-14).

In subarachnoid hemorrhage, blood appears in the subarachnoid space, which is located between the pia mater and the arachnoid mater. Blood may also appear in the ventricular system (intraventricular hemorrhage), as this is connected to the subarachnoid space. Subarachnoid hemorrhage is most commonly caused by leakage of blood from an aneurysm, but may also be caused by trauma.

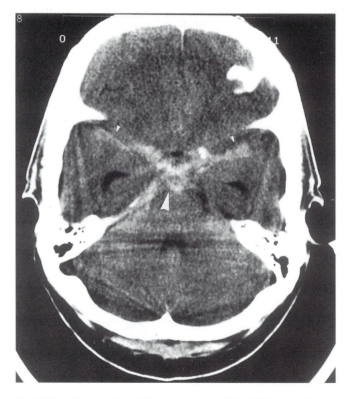

Fig.9-13: Subarachnoid hemorrhage. This CT image taken at the *Star* level demonstrates bright blood in the suprasellar cistern (large arrowhead) and in the Sylvian fissures (small arrowheads).

In this entity, there is blood in the epidural space, which is located between the dura mater and the skull. It often caused by an arterial tear (especially the middle meningeal artery). It is usually caused by significant trauma and is often associated with skull fractures.

B. Trauma (3 B's)

In head trauma, three primary injuries may occur. These may be remembered by the **three B's**, which include: a **B**leed inside the skull (intracranial hemorrhage), a **B**ruise within the brain (cerebral contusion) or a **B**reak in the skull bones (fracture).

1. Bleeds (hemorrhages)

Intracranial hemorrhage is commonly associated with trauma. For a more complete discussion of intracranial hemorrhages, refer to the previous section.

2. Bruises (contusions)

A contusion is an area of bruised brain. On CT scan, it appears as a hypodense area (dark area compared to brain tissue). It most frequently occurs in the anterior portion of the

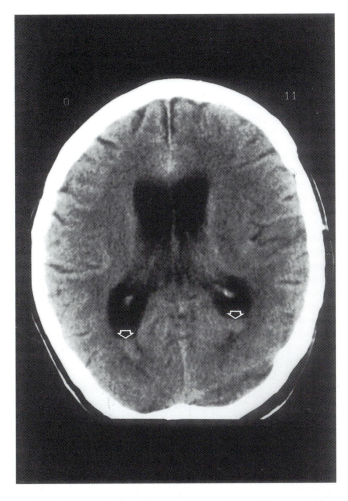

Fig.9-14: Intraventricular hemorrhage. This CT image taken at the *Worms* level demonstrates a small amount of blood in the occipital horns, the most dependent area of the lateral ventricles (open arrows).

3. Subdural

On CT scan, this appears as a bright "moon crescent" between the brain and the skull (Fig.9-15). It crosses suture lines but never crosses dural reflections (i.e. falx cerebri and the tentorium).

In this entity there is blood in the subdural space, which is located between the dura mater and the arachnoid mater. It is most often caused by a venous tear, and occurs often in elderly patients. It frequently occurs secondary to minor trauma (half of the patients cannot even recall the injury that caused the bleed). It is relatively rare to find a skull fracture when a subdural hematoma is present.

4. Epidural

On CT scan, this has the appearance of a biconvex white lens, located between the brain and the skull (Fig.9-16). Unlike the subdural hematoma, the epidural hematoma may cross dural reflections, but does not cross suture lines.

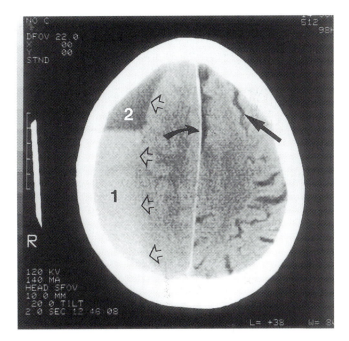

Fig.9-15: Acute and chronic subdural hemorrhage. This CT image taken at the *Coffee Bean* level, demonstrates a crescent shaped abnormality on the right side of the patient consistent with a subdural hematoma (open arrows). The bright area of the crescent represents acute hemorrhage (1), whereas the dark portion of the hematoma represents chronic hemorrhage (2). Notice also that there is a mild mass effect. No sulci are seen on the side of the hematoma, while sulci are easily visualized in the contralateral hemisphere (straight black arrow). Notice also that the bright falx is bowed away from the abnormality (curved black arrow).

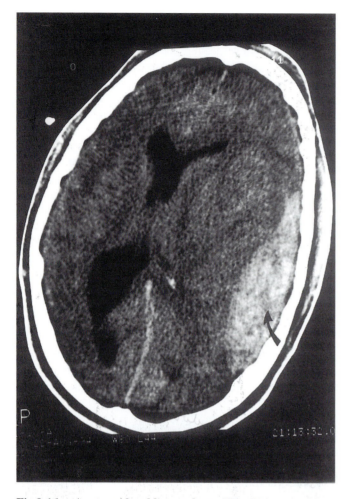

Fig.9-16: **Acute epidural hemorrhage.** This CT image taken at the *Mr. Sad* level demonstrates a lens-shaped bright abnormality of the left side of the patient (curved black arrow). There is also a marked mass effect on the surrounding brain.

temporal lobes and in the inferior portion of the frontal lobes. There may also be bright blood in a bruised area (hemorrhagic contusion).

3. Breaks (fractures)

All the previously seen CT images were photographed at a "brain window." This just means that the pictures are designed to see the densities of the brain really well. The problem is that on these images, the bony structures appear very white and little detail is seen within them. To best see fractures, CT images can be photographed at a "bone window." On these images, the high density bones are well seen while the brain is barely visible (Fig.9-17).

Fractures have the appearance of a dark line running through the white-colored skull (Fig.9-17). These should not be confused with suture lines, which always appear bilaterally in approximately the same location.

Skull base fractures present a special problem because the anatomy of this region is complex. Simply, if there is air in-

side the skull, and especially near the base, and no other reason exists to account for this finding (i.e., recent neurosurgery), then there is likely a skull base fracture.

C. Stroke

1. Ischemic (dark)

On CT scans, this entity may have a normal appearance for the first 12 hours. The first manifestations of an infarct are subtle and include a white clot in one of the vessels, loss of normal gray-white differentiation, and sulcal flattening (*effacement*). Thereafter, the appearance often progresses to a wedge-shaped dark area, extending to the edge of the brain, involving both the gray and white matter (Fig.9-18).

Infarction occurs when an area of brain gets insufficient blood perfusion and dies. Causes of stroke include atherosclerosis, emboli, low cardiac output and vasospasm. Infarcts may be very small and round. These are lacunar infarcts and are often located in the deep brain (basal ganglia, thalamus, internal capsule and the brain stem; Fig.9-18).

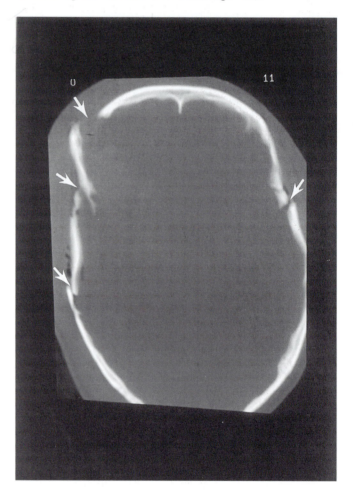

Fig.9-17. Skull fractures. This CT image has been taken at a *bone window,* which clearly displays the skull bones but barely displays the brain. In this image, several skull fractures can be identified (white arrows).

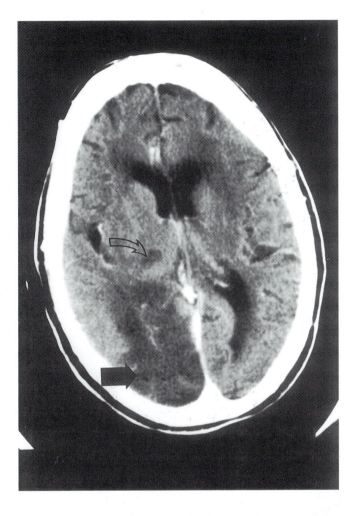

Fig.9-18: Right posterior cerebral artery territory stroke and right thalamic lacuna. This CT image taken at the *Mr. Sad* level shows an abnormal dark area in the right occipital lobe consistent with a posterior cerebral artery territory infarct (large black arrow). A second smaller abnormal dark area is seen in the right thalamus consistent with a right thalamic lacunar infarct (curved empty arrow).

As described in the vascular anatomy section, different areas of the brain are supplied by different arteries. Therefore, by determining where the abnormality is located, one may deduct which vessel is the culprit.

2. Acute hemorrhagic (bright)

On CT scan, this entity appears as an abnormal area of bright blood within the brain tissue. Approximately one fifth of patients with a clinical presentation of stroke have a hemorrhagic stroke. Anticoagulant and thrombolytic medication may be indicated in ischemic stroke. When given to patients with hemorrhagic strokes, they may be deadly. Because of this, it is important to rule out hemorrhage via CT before treating the patient.

D. Mass effect

Several space occupying lesions may appear within the brain, including abscesses, tumors and hematomas. When these occur, the brain may be pushed away, causing loss of normal symmetry between the two cerebral hemispheres. If severe enough, parts of the brain may slide (*herniate*) under either the dural reflections (*falx, tentorium*) or down the foramen magnum of the skull. There are three types of herniation: subfalcine, transtentorial, and tonsillar herniation.

1. Subfalcine herniation

Subfalcine herniation occurs when some brain tissue or a lateral ventricle slides under the falx cerebri towards the opposite side (Fig.9-19). On the film, when the septum pellucidum is bowed to one side because of mass effect, there is subfalcine herniation.

2. Uncal herniation

Uncal herniation occurs when some brain tissue (*uncus*) slides under the tentorium towards the superior surface of the cerebellum. On CT scan, the star (*suprasellar cistern*)

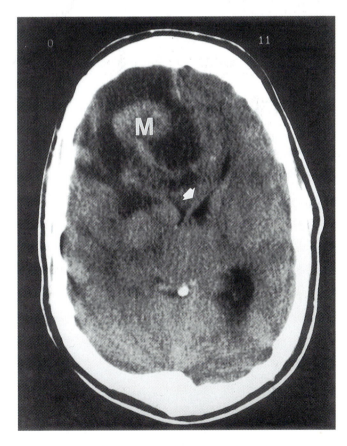

Fig.9-19: Subfalcine herniation. This CT image taken at the *Mr. Sad* level shows a mass (M) in the right hemisphere, which is causing displacement of the septum pellucidum to the left (arrow).

may be deformed. In addition, the brainstem is pushed away by the mass. Because the cerebellum is attached to the brainstem, the cerebellum is also pushed away from the mass. Lastly, there may be small bright areas of hemorrhage in the anterior midbrain (called *Duret hemorrhages*), or cerebral dark infarcts in the posterior cerebral artery territory.

3. Tonsilar herniation

This entity is difficult to visualize on CT scan. It occurs when the cerebellar tonsils slip through the foramen magnum out of the skull. Obviously, this represents bad news!

E. Hydrocephalus

Hydrocephalus occurs when either all (*communicating hydrocephalus*) or part (*non-communicating hydrocephalus*) of the ventricular system is dilated.

1. Non-communicating (normal 4th ventricle)

This type is secondary to an obstruction of the ventricular system (foramen of Monro, 3rd ventricle, aqueduct of Sylvius or 4th ventricle). It results in dilatation of the system proximal to the obstruction. The choroid plexi in the lateral ventricles continue making CSF oblivious to the obstruction. Pressure within the lateral ventricle pushes the brain tissue against the skull and causes sulcal effacement or flattening (similar to an old man squishing his face in a window, resulting in wrinkle effacement). Often, the pressure is great enough within the ventricles so that some CSF spreads into the brain tissue around the ventricles, through the ventricular wall (the *ependyma*).

Therefore the CT scan findings may include sulci effacement, transependymal spread of CSF, and dilation of all the ventricles proximal to the level of blockage (Fig.9-20). Therefore, if the blockage is between the third and the fourth ventricle, the 4th ventricle will be of normal size. If the blockage is located between the lateral ventricles and the third ventricle, both the third and the fourth ventricle will be normal. Common causes of non-communicating hydrocephalus include tumors and congenital defects.

2. Communicating hydrocephalus (dilated 4th ventricle)

In this type, the obstruction occurs distal to the fourth ventricle (i.e. in the subarachnoid space or in arachnoid granulation tissue where CSF is resorbed). The CT findings

are similar to the above, except that the entire ventricular system, including the 4th ventricle, is dilated. This entity is often caused by *meningitis,* subarachnoid hemorrhage and trauma.

3. Ex vacuo hydrocephalus (cerebral atrophy)

Cerebral atrophy occurs when there is less brain tissue than normal. This is more commonly seen with old age. Because there is less brain, the ventricles fill the increased space and appear enlarged. In contrast with other types of hydrocephalus, the cerebral sulci are bigger instead of being squished against the skull. There is no blockage and no increased pressure in the ventricular system. Ex vacuo hydrocephalus is of no clinical significance and is not to be confused with other types of hydrocephalus.

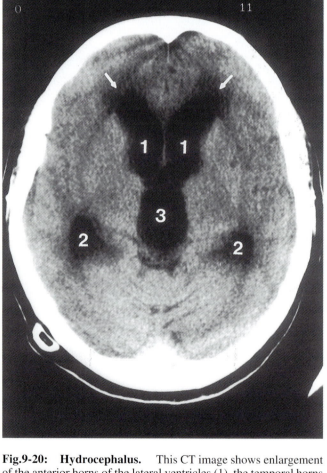

Fig.9-20: Hydrocephalus. This CT image shows enlargement of the anterior horns of the lateral ventricles (1), the temporal horns of the lateral ventricles (2) and the third ventricle (3). The abnormal dark areas adjacent to the frontal horn represent transependymal CSF spread (white arrows). Note that no sulci are visible at the brain's surface.

Index